UNDERGROUND CLINICAL VIGNETTES

Pathophysiology I: Pulmonary, Ob/Gyn, ENT, Hem/Onc

FIFTH EDITION

Underground Clinical Vignettes

Pathophysiology I: Pulmonary, Ob/Gyn, ENT, Hem/Onc

FIFTH EDITION

Todd A. Swanson, M.D., Ph.D.
Resident in Radiation Oncology
William Beaumont Hospital
Royal Oak, Michigan

Sandra I. Kim, M.D., Ph.D.
Resident in Internal Medicine
Beth Israel Deaconess Medical Center
Harvard Medical School
Boston, Massachusetts

Olga E. Flomin, M.D.
Resident in Obstetrics and Gynecology
William Beaumont Hospital
Royal Oak, Michigan

 Wolters Kluwer | Lippincott Williams & Wilkins
Health

Philadelphia • Baltimore • New York • London
Buenos Aires • Hong Kong • Sydney • Tokyo

Acquisitions Editor: Nancy Anastasi Duffy
Developmental Editor: Kathleen H. Scogna
Managing Editor: Nancy Hoffmann
Marketing Manager: Jennifer Kuklinski
Associate Production Manager: Kevin P. Johnson
Creative Director: Doug Smock
Compositor: International Typesetting and Composition
Printer: R.R. Donnelley & Son's - Crawfordsville

**WB
18.2
P2971
2008**

First Edition, 2001 Blackwell Publishing Inc.
Second Edition, 2003 Blackwell Publishing Inc.
Third Edition, 2005 Blackwell Publishing Inc.
Fourth Edition, 2005 Blackwell Publishing Inc.

Library of Congress Cataloging-in-Publication Data

Swanson, Todd A.
  Pathophysiology. I, Pulmonary, ob/gyn, ENT, hem/onc / Todd Swanson, Sandra Kim, Olga E. Flomin. — 5th ed.
      p. ; cm. — (Underground clinical vignettes)
  Rev. ed. of: Pathophysiology / Tao Le . . . [et al.]. 4th ed. c2005.
  Includes bibliographical references and index.
  ISBN-13: 978-0-7817-6465-0
  ISBN-10: 0-7817-6465-3
  1. Physiology, Pathological—Case studies.
2. Physicians—Licenses—Examinations—Study guides.   I. Kim, Sandra.
II. Flomin, Olga E.   III. Pathophysiology.   IV. Title.   V. Title: Pulmonary, ob/gyn, ENT, hem/onc.   VI. Series.
  [DNLM: 1. Clinical Medicine—Case Reports.   2. Clinical Medicine—Problems and Exercises.   WB 18.2 S972p 2006]
    RB113.B459 2006
    616.07'076—dc22

                                                              2006100528

dedication
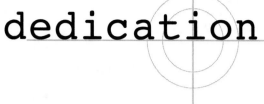

For T.M.

preface

First published in 1999, the *Underground Clinical Vignettes* (UCV) series has provided thousands of students with a highly effective review tool as they prepare for medical exams, particularly the USMLE Step 1 and 2 exams. Designed as a quick study guide, each UCV book contains patient-centered clinical cases that highlight a range of medical diagnoses.

With this new edition of UCV, we have incorporated feedback from medical students across the country to provide updated cases with expanded treatment and discussion sections. A new two-page format enables readers to formulate an initial diagnosis prior to reading the answer, while the added differential diagnosis section encourages critical thinking about comparable cases. The inclusion of relevant MRI images, x-rays, and photographs allows students to more readily visualize the physical presentation of each case. Breakout boxes, tables, and algorithms have been added, along with all new Board format QAs, making this edition of UCV an ideal source of information for exam review, classroom discussion, or clinical rotations.

The clinical vignettes in this series are designed to give added emphasis to pathogenesis, epidemiology, management, and complications. Although each case tends to present all the signs, symptoms, and diagnostic findings for a particular illness, patients generally will not present with such a "complete" picture either clinically or on a medical examination. Cases are not meant to simulate a potential real patient or an exam vignette.

Access to LWW's online companion site, ThePoint, will be offered as a premium with the purchase of the Underground Clinical Vignettes Step 1 bundle. Benefits include an online test link and additional new Board format questions covering all UCV subject areas.

We hope you will find the UCV series informative and useful. We welcome any feedback, suggestions, or corrections you have about this series. Please contact us at LWW.com/medstudent.

contributors

Series Editors

Todd A. Swanson, M.D., Ph.D.
Resident in Radiation Oncology
William Beaumont Hospital
Royal Oak, Michigan

Sandra I. Kim, M.D., Ph.D.
Resident in Internal Medicine
Beth Israel Deaconess Medical Center
Harvard Medical School
Boston, Massachusetts

Series Contributors

Olga E. Flomin, M.D.
Resident in Obstetrics and Gynecology
William Beaumont Hospital
Royal Oak, Michigan

Medina C. Kushen, M.D.
Resident in Neurosurgery
University of Chicago Hospitals
Chicago, Illinois

Marc J. Glucksman, Ph.D.
Professor of Biochemistry and Molecular Biology
Director, Midwest Proteome Center and
Co-Director, Rosalind Franklin Structural Biology Laboratories
Rosalind Franklin University of Medicine and Science
The Chicago Medical School
North Chicago, Illinois

acknowledgments

Thanks to Dr. Alvaro Martinez, Dr. Larry Kestin and the entire radiation oncology program at William Beaumont Hospital for allowing the flexibility to work on this project during an already vigorous residency training program.

— Todd A. Swanson

Thanks to Todd for his work on this series.

— Sandra I. Kim

abbreviations

ABPA	allergic bronchopulmonary aspergillosis	CABG	coronary artery bypass grafting
ACA	anticardiolipin antibody	CAD	coronary artery disease
ACE	angiotensin-converting enzyme	CaEDTA	calcium edetate
ACL	anterior cruciate ligament	CALLA	common acute lymphoblastic leukemia antigen
ACTH	adrenocorticotropic hormone	cAMP	cyclic adenosine monophosphate
AD	adjustment disorder	C-ANCA	cytoplasmic antineutrophil cyto-
ADA	adenosine deaminase		plasmic antibody
ADD	attention deficit disorder	CBC	complete blood count
ADH	antidiuretic hormone	CBD	common bile duct
ADHD	attention deficit hyperactivity disorder	CCU	cardiac care unit
		CD	cluster of differentiation
ADP	adenosine diphosphate	2-CdA	2-chlorodeoxyadenosine
AFO	ankle-foot orthosis	CEA	carcinoembryonic antigen
AFP	α-fetoprotein	CFTR	cystic fibrosis transmembrane conductance regulator
AIDS	acquired immunodeficiency syndrome		
		cGMP	cyclic guanosine monophos- phate
ALL	acute lymphocytic leukemia		
ALS	amyotrophic lateral sclerosis	CHF	congestive heart failure
ALT	alanine aminotransferase	CK	creatine kinase
AML	acute myelogenous leukemia	CK-MB	creatine kinase, MB fraction
ANA	antinuclear antibody	CLL	chronic lymphocytic leukemia
Angio	angiography	CML	chronic myelogenous leukemia
AP	anteroposterior	CMV	cytomegalovirus
APKD	adult polycystic kidney disease	CN	cranial nerve
aPTT	activated partial thromboplastin time	CNS	central nervous system
		COPD	chronic obstructive pulmonary disease
ARDS	adult respiratory distress syn- drome		
		COX	cyclooxygenase
5-ASA	5-aminosalicylic acid	CP	cerebellopontine
ASCA	antibodies to Saccharomyces cerevisiae	CPAP	continuous positive airway pressure
ASO	antistreptolysin O	CPK	creatine phosphokinase
AST	aspartate aminotransferase	CPPD	calcium pyrophosphate dihydrate
ATLL	adult T-cell leukemia/lymphoma	CPR	cardiopulmonary resuscitation
ATPase	adenosine triphosphatase	CREST	calcinosis, Raynaud's phenome- non, esophageal involvement, sclerodactyly, telangiectasia (syndrome)
AV	arteriovenous, atrioventricular		
AZT	azidothymidine (zidovudine)		
BAL	British antilewisite (dimercaprol)		
BCG	bacille Calmette-Guérin	CRP	C-reactive protein
BE	barium enema	CSF	cerebrospinal fluid
BP	blood pressure	CSOM	chronic suppurative otitis media
BPH	benign prostatic hypertrophy	CT	cardiac transplant, computed tomography
BUN	blood urea nitrogen		

CVA	cerebrovascular accident	ER	emergency room
CXR	chest x-ray	ERCP	endoscopic retrograde cholan-giopancreatography
d4T	didehydrodeoxythymidine (stavudine)		
		ERT	estrogen replacement therapy
DCS	decompression sickness	ESR	erythrocyte sedimentation rate
DDH	developmental dysplasia of the hip	ETEC	enterotoxigenic *E. coli*
		EtOH	ethanol
ddl	dideoxyinosine (didanosine)	FAP	familial adenomatous polyposis
DES	diethylstilbestrol	FEV_1	forced expiratory volume in 1 second
DEXA	dual-energy x-ray absorptiometry		
		FH	familial hypercholesterolemia
DHEAS	dehydroepiandrosterone sulfate	FNA	fine-needle aspiration
DIC	disseminated intravascular coagulation	FSH	follicle-stimulating hormone
		FTA-ABS	fluorescent treponemal antibody absorption test
DIF	direct immunofluorescence		
DIP	distal interphalangeal (joint)	FVC	forced vital capacity
DKA	diabetic ketoacidosis	G6PD	glucose-6-phosphate dehydrogenase
DL_{CO}	diffusing capacity of carbon monoxide		
		GABA	gamma-aminobutyric acid
DMSA	2,3-dimercaptosuccinic acid	GERD	gastroesophageal reflux disease
DNA	deoxyribonucleic acid		
DNase	deoxyribonuclease	GFR	glomerular filtration rate
2,3-DPG	2,3-diphosphoglycerate	GGT	gamma-glutamyltransferase
dsDNA	double-stranded DNA	GH	growth hormone
DSM	Diagnostic and Statistical Manual	GI	gastrointestinal
dsRNA	double-stranded RNA	GnRH	gonadotropin-releasing hormone
DTP	diphtheria, tetanus, pertussis (vaccine)		
		GU	genitourinary
DTPA	diethylenetriamine-penta-acetic acid	GVHD	graft-versus-host disease
		HAART	highly active antiretroviral therapy
DTs	delirium tremens		
DVT	deep venous thrombosis	HAV	hepatitis A virus
EBV	Epstein-Barr virus	Hb	hemoglobin
ECG	electrocardiography	HbA-1C	hemoglobin A-1C
Echo	echocardiography	HBsAg	hepatitis B surface antigen
ECM	erythema chronicum migrans	HBV	hepatitis B virus
ECT	electroconvulsive therapy	hCG	human chorionic gonadotropin
EEG	electroencephalography	HCO_3	bicarbonate
EF	ejection fraction, elongation factor	Hct	hematocrit
		HCV	hepatitis C virus
EGD	esophagogastroduodenoscopy	HDL	high-density lipoprotein
EHEC	enterohemorrhagic *E. coli*	HDL-C	high-density lipoprotein-cholesterol
EIA	enzyme immunoassay		
ELISA	enzyme-linked immunosorbent assay	HEENT	head, eyes, ears, nose, and throat (exam)
EM	electron microscopy	HELLP	hemolysis, elevated LFTs, low platelets (syndrome)
EMG	electromyography		
ENT	ears, nose, and throat	HFMD	hand, foot, and mouth disease
EPVE	early prosthetic valve endocarditis	HGPRT	hypoxanthine-guanine phospho-ribosyltransferase

5-HIAA	5-hydroxyindoleacetic acid	LES	lower esophageal sphincter
HIDA	hepato-iminodiacetic acid (scan)	LFTs	liver function tests
HIV	human immunodeficiency virus	LH	luteinizing hormone
HLA	human leukocyte antigen	LMN	lower motor neuron
HMG-CoA	hydroxymethylglutaryl-coenzyme A	LP	lumbar puncture
		LPVE	late prosthetic valve endocarditis
HMP	hexose monophosphate		
HPI	history of present illness	L/S	lecithin-sphingomyelin (ratio)
HPV	human papillomavirus	LSD	lysergic acid diethylamide
HR	heart rate	LT	labile toxin
HRIG	human rabies immune globulin	LV	left ventricular
HRS	hepatorenal syndrome	LVH	left ventricular hypertrophy
HRT	hormone replacement therapy	Lytes	electrolytes
HSG	hysterosalpingography	Mammo	mammography
HSV	herpes simplex virus	MAO	monoamine oxidase (inhibitor)
HTLV	human T-cell leukemia virus	MCP	metacarpophalangeal (joint)
HUS	hemolytic-uremic syndrome	MCTD	mixed connective tissue disorder
HVA	homovanillic acid		
ICP	intracranial pressure	MCV	mean corpuscular volume
ICU	intensive care unit	MEN	multiple endocrine neoplasia
ID/CC	identification and chief complaint	MI	myocardial infarction
		MIBG	meta-iodobenzylguanidine (radioisotope)
IDDM	insulin-dependent diabetes mellitus		
		MMR	measles, mumps, rubella (vaccine)
IFA	immunofluorescent antibody		
Ig	immunoglobulin	MPGN	membranoproliferative glomerulonephritis
IGF	insulin-like growth factor		
IHSS	idiopathic hypertrophic subaortic stenosis	MPS	mucopolysaccharide
		MPTP	1-methyl-4-phenyl-tetrahydropyridine
IM	intramuscular		
IMA	inferior mesenteric artery	MR	magnetic resonance (imaging)
INH	isoniazid	mRNA	messenger ribonucleic acid
INR	International Normalized Ratio	MRSA	methicillin-resistant S. aureus
IP_3	inositol 1,4,5-triphosphate	MTP	metatarsophalangeal (joint)
IPF	idiopathic pulmonary fibrosis	NAD	nicotinamide adenine dinucleotide
ITP	idiopathic thrombocytopenic purpura		
		NADP	nicotinamide adenine dinucleotide phosphate
IUD	intrauterine device		
IV	intravenous	NADPH	reduced nicotinamide adenine dinucleotide phosphate
IVC	inferior vena cava		
IVIG	intravenous immunoglobulin	NF	neurofibromatosis
IVP	intravenous pyelography	NIDDM	non-insulin-dependent diabetes mellitus
JRA	juvenile rheumatoid arthritis		
JVP	jugular venous pressure	NNRTI	non-nucleoside reverse transcriptase inhibitor
KOH	potassium hydroxide		
KUB	kidney, ureter, bladder	NO	nitric oxide
LCM	lymphocytic choriomeningitis	NPO	nil per os (nothing by mouth)
LDH	lactate dehydrogenase	NSAID	nonsteroidal anti-inflammatory drug
LDL	low-density lipoprotein		
LE	lupus erythematosus (cell)	Nuc	nuclear medicine

NYHA	New York Heart Association	PPH	primary postpartum hemorrhage
OB	obstetric		
OCD	obsessive-compulsive disorder	PRA	panel reactive antibody
OCPs	oral contraceptive pills	PROM	premature rupture of membranes
OR	operating room		
PA	posteroanterior	PSA	prostate-specific antigen
PABA	para-aminobenzoic acid	PSS	progressive systemic sclerosis
PAN	polyarteritis nodosa	PT	prothrombin time
P-ANCA	perinuclear antineutrophil cytoplasmic antibody	PTH	parathyroid hormone
		PTSD	post-traumatic stress disorder
Pao_2	partial pressure of oxygen in arterial blood	PTT	partial thromboplastin time
		PUVA	psoralen ultraviolet A
PAS	periodic acid Schiff	PVC	premature ventricular contraction
PAT	paroxysmal atrial tachycardia		
PBS	peripheral blood smear	RA	rheumatoid arthritis
Pco_2	partial pressure of carbon dioxide	RAIU	radioactive iodine uptake
		RAST	radioallergosorbent test
PCOM	posterior communicating (artery)	RBC	red blood cell
		REM	rapid eye movement
PCOS	polycystic ovarian syndrome	RES	reticuloendothelial system
PCP	phencyclidine	RFFIT	rapid fluorescent focus inhibition test
PCR	polymerase chain reaction		
PCT	porphyria cutanea tarda	RFTs	renal function tests
PCTA	percutaneous coronary transluminal angioplasty	RHD	rheumatic heart disease
		RNA	ribonucleic acid
PCV	polycythemia vera	RNP	ribonucleoprotein
PDA	patent ductus arteriosus	RPR	rapid plasma reagin
PDGF	platelet-derived growth factor	RR	respiratory rate
PE	physical exam	RSV	respiratory syncytial virus
PEFR	peak expiratory flow rate	RUQ	right upper quadrant
PEG	polyethylene glycol	RV	residual volume
PEPCK	phosphoenolpyruvate carboxykinase	Sao_2	oxygen saturation in arterial blood
PET	positron emission tomography	SBFT	small bowel follow-through
PFTs	pulmonary function tests	SCC	squamous cell carcinoma
PID	pelvic inflammatory disease	SCID	severe combined immunodeficiency
PIP	proximal interphalangeal (joint)		
PKU	phenylketonuria	SERM	selective estrogen receptor modulator
PMDD	premenstrual dysphoric disorder		
		SGOT	serum glutamic-oxaloacetic transaminase
PML	progressive multifocal leukoencephalopathy		
		SIADH	syndrome of inappropriate antidiuretic hormone
PMN	polymorphonuclear (leukocyte)		
PNET	primitive neuroectodermal tumor	SIDS	sudden infant death syndrome
		SLE	systemic lupus erythematosus
PNH	paroxysmal nocturnal hemoglobinuria	SMA	superior mesenteric artery
		SSPE	subacute sclerosing panencephalitis
Po_2	partial pressure of oxygen		
PPD	purified protein derivative (of tuberculosis)	SSRI	selective serotonin reuptake inhibitor

ST	stable toxin	UA	urinalysis
STD	sexually transmitted disease	UDCA	ursodeoxycholic acid
T2W	T2-weighted (MRI)	UGI	upper GI
T_3	triiodothyronine	UPPP	uvulopalatopharyngoplasty
T_4	thyroxine	URI	upper respiratory infection
TAH-BSO	total abdominal hysterectomy–bilateral salpingo-oophorectomy	US	ultrasound
		UTI	urinary tract infection
		UV	ultraviolet
TB	tuberculosis	VDRL	Venereal Disease Research Laboratory
TCA	tricyclic antidepressant		
TCC	transitional cell carcinoma	VIN	vulvar intraepithelial neoplasia
TDT	terminal deoxytransferase	VIP	vasoactive intestinal polypeptide
TFTs	thyroid function tests		
TGF	transforming growth factor	VLDL	very low density lipoprotein
THC	tetrahydrocannabinol	VMA	vanillylmandelic acid
TIA	transient ischemic attack	V/Q	ventilation/perfusion (ratio)
TLC	total lung capacity	VRE	vancomycin-resistant enterococcus
TMP-SMX	trimethoprim-sulfamethoxazole		
tPA	tissue plasminogen activator	VS	vital signs
TP-HA	*Treponema pallidum* hemagglutination assay	VSD	ventricular septal defect
		vWF	von Willebrand's factor
TPP	thiamine pyrophosphate	VZV	varicella-zoster virus
TRAP	tartrate-resistant acid phosphatase	WAGR	Wilms' tumor, aniridia, genitourinary abnormalities, mental retardation (syndrome)
tRNA	transfer ribonucleic acid		
TSH	thyroid-stimulating hormone	WBC	white blood cell
TSS	toxic shock syndrome	WHI	Women's Health Initiative
TTP	thrombotic thrombocytopenic purpura	WPW	Wolff-Parkinson-White syndrome
TURP	transurethral resection of the prostate	XR	x-ray
		ZN	Ziehl-Neelsen (stain)
TXA	thromboxane A		

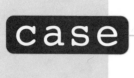

ID/CC A 45-year-old white female is rushed to the OR because of **shock** due to postoperative bleeding; during intubation, she **vomits and aspirates** that day's breakfast.

HPI She had undergone a cholecystectomy 2 days before and had presented with postoperative bleeding requiring surgical exploration.

PE VS: **tachycardia; tachypnea; fever; hypotension.** PE: **central cyanosis;** warm, moist skin; **intercostal retraction; inspiratory crepitant rales** heard over both lung fields.

Labs CBC/PBS: marked **leukocytosis** with neutrophilia; fragmented RBCs; thrombocytopenia. ABGs: **severe hypoxemia with no improvement on 100% oxygen;** ratio of arterial Po_2 to inspired fraction of O_2 <200. Increased BUN and creatinine; increased AST and ALT.

Imaging CXR: typical **diffuse and symmetric parahilar ("batwing" pattern) alveolar filling** process suggestive of **noncardiogenic pulmonary edema.**

Gross Pathology Formation of **hyaline membranes** with proteinaceous deposits in alveoli; **pulmonary edema** with red, heavy lungs which, combined with **widespread atelectasis,** produce **stiff lung** with fibrosis.

Micro Pathology Endothelial and alveolocapillary damage with edema, hyaline membrane formation, and inflammatory infiltrate; **loss of surfactant** with fibroblast activity in later stages.

1

case 1

Acute Respiratory Distress Syndrome (ARDS)

Differential

Altitude Sickness
Congestive Heart Failure
Pulmonary Edema
Pneumonia

Discussion

Adult respiratory distress syndrome is a condition that is associated with **high mortality**; it is caused by gram-negative **sepsis, massive trauma**; burns, disseminated intravascular coagulation (DIC), acute pancreatitis, narcotic overdose, and near drowning. It is characterized by diffuse alveolar capillary injury, which leads to an increase in vascular permeability and pulmonary edema. The increased permeability results in leakage of inflammatory cells into the interstitium and alveolar spaces. Damage to the **type II pneumocytes that produce surfactant** occur, resulting in collapse of alveoli with impaired gas exchange. **Waxy hyaline membranes** consisting of **fibrin-rich edema fluid** and **necrotic cells** form further impairing gas exchange. Ultimately, ventilation perfusion (V/Q) mismatching occurs.

Treatment

Mechanical ventilation with moderate to high levels of positive end-expiratory pressure **(PEEP)**; antibiotics, steroids, close monitoring of hemodynamic function.

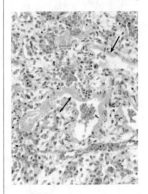

Figure 1-1. Waxy hyaline membranes consisting of fibrin-rich edema fluid and necrotic cells.

ID/CC	A **65-year-old male** presents with **progressively increasing cough and dyspnea** on exertion.
HPI	He is a **retired naval shipyard worker** and has a nearly **100-pack-year smoking** history.
PE	VS: normal. PE: grade II **clubbing;** fine crackles auscultated bilaterally over lung bases.
Labs	CBC: normal. PFTs: mixed obstructive and restrictive disease pattern; reduced DL_{CO}.
Imaging	CXR: irregular linear, **interstitial infiltrates** in lower lobes with circumscribed radiopaque densities (PLEURAL PLAQUES). CT (high resolution): posterior and lateral pleura thickened with **calcified plaques** seen bilaterally.
Gross Pathology	Diffuse pulmonary **interstitial fibrosis** with **bilateral pleural calcification** and thickening and involvement of the diaphragm.
Micro Pathology	Calcium-containing dense pleural opacities and plaques of collagen; **ferruginous bodies.**

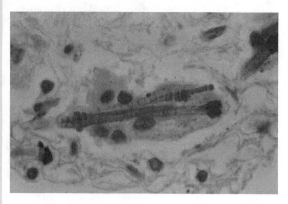

Figure 2-1. Ferruginous body.

3

case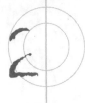

Asbestosis

Differential

Pneumoconiosis

Dermatomyositis

Hypersensitivity Pneumonitis

Idiopathic Pulmonary Fibrosis

Sarcoidosis

Silicosis

Discussion

Microscopic exam of sputum reveals **golden-brown beaded rods** (ASBESTOS/FERRUGINOUS BODIES) composed of asbestos fibers coated with an iron-containing proteinaceous material. Although classic in the presentation, these are not required for the diagnosis, as normal people may have such findings. Prolonged exposure to asbestos in significantly cumulative doses results in **pulmonary parenchymal scarring.** This process is self-perpetuating, but cessation of exposure may slow disease progression. Complications include **bronchogenic carcinoma, malignant mesothelioma, cor pulmonale,** and death; smoking and asbestos exposure **synergistically** increase cancer risk.

Treatment

Supportive and symptomatic treatment (oxygen, bronchodilators, antibiotics); **prevention of further exposure; smoking cessation;** counseling regarding **high risk** of **bronchogenic carcinoma** and **malignant mesothelioma.**

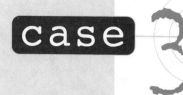

case

ID/CC A 10-year-old girl is brought into the ER in **acute respiratory distress**.

HPI The patient is known to be **allergic** to cats and pollen; her mother states that she had a **recent URI**. She also complains of a history of moderate **intermittent dyspnea that is exacerbated by exercise**.

PE VS: no fever; **tachypnea** (RR 32); BP: normal. PE: inspiratory and **expiratory wheezes** (due to bronchoconstriction, small airway inflammation); boggy and pale nasal mucosa; **accessory muscle** use during breathing; enlarged chest AP diameter; **hyperresonant** to percussion.

Labs ABGs: primary respiratory alkalosis (hyperventilation). CBC: **eosinophilia** (13%). PFTs: low FEV_1/FVC.

Imaging CXR: hyperinflation with flattened diaphragms (increased residual volume due to **air trapping**); peribronchial cuffing.

Gross Pathology **Hyperinflation** with air trapping in alveoli; **plugs of inspissated mucus**; edema of mucosal lining.

Micro Pathology Inflammatory infiltrate of bronchial epithelium, mainly eosinophilic; plugging of airways **with thickened mucus** (CURSCHMANN'S SPIRALS); hypertrophy of mucous glands; elongated rhomboid crystals derived from eosinophil cytoplasm (CHARCOT–LEYDEN CRYSTALS); hyperplasia of smooth muscle of bronchi.

case 3

Bronchial Asthma

Differential
: α_1-antitrypsin Deficiency
Bronchiolitis
Churg-Strauss Syndrome
Foreign Body Aspiration
Gastroesophageal Reflux Disease (GERD)
Congestive Heart Failure (Cardiac Asthma)
Allergic Bronchopulmonary Aspergillosis

Discussion
: Bronchial asthma is characterized by **hyperreactivity of the airways** and obstruction due to bronchospasm, edema, and mucus. It is also known as **reactive airway disease.**

Treatment
: Nebulized bronchodilators, parenteral steroids, and ventilatory support for acute exacerbations; inhaled bronchodilators and steroids for chronic, persistent symptoms; mast cell stabilizers such as cromolyn and leukotriene inhibitors such as zafirlukast for prophylaxis.

■ TABLE 3-1 ASTHMA SEVERITY

Severity	Symptoms	Treatment
Mild Intermittent	<2 times per week	Short acting adrenergic inhalers
Mild Persistent	>2 times per week	Short acting adrenergic inhalers + low dose inhaled steroids or + Cromolyn or + Leukotriene modifier
Moderate Persistent	Daily, interferes with activities	Short acting adrenergic inhalers + moderate dose inhaled steroids Or + low dose inhaled steroids and long acting adrenergic agonist Or + low dose inhaled steroids and Leukotriene modifier)
Severe Persistent	Continual, limits activity, frequent exacerbations	High-dose inhaled steroids and Long-acting adrenergic agonist

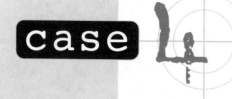

ID/CC A 50-year-old white male develops a **fever 24 hours after surgery.**

HPI He underwent an emergency **laparotomy** for a perforated peptic ulcer without any intraoperative or immediate postoperative complications.

PE VS: **fever**; BP normal; **tachypnea; tachycardia.** PE: no cyanosis; **scattered rales** and **decreased breath sounds;** no calf tenderness; no hematoma or discharge from wound; no inflammation of IV line veins; no urinary symptoms.

Labs ABGs: mild **hypoxemia.** CBC: slight neutrophilic leukocytosis. Blood and sputum culture sterile. ECG: sinus tachycardia.

Imaging CXR: **dense opacity in left lower lobe** (collapsed lobe) with elevation of right hemidiaphragm (due to volume loss).

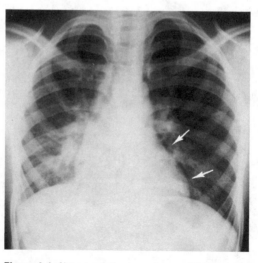

Figure 4-1. Note area of apparent consolidation in the right paratracheal region (arrows).

7

case 4

Atelectasis—Postoperative

Differential

Asbestosis

Hypersensitivity Pneumonitis

Bronchogenic Carcinoma

Pneumonia

Idiopathic Pulmonary Fibrosis

Pulmonary Embolism

Discussion

Postoperative atelectasis is the most common cause of postoperative fever in the first 48 hours; alveolar collapse is produced by occlusion due to viscid secretions favored by recumbency, hypoventilation, and oversedation. Other causes of postoperative fever, usually seen later in the postoperative period, include UTI, IV catheter infection, deep venous thrombosis, wound infection, and drug reactions.

Treatment

Chest physiotherapy (incentive spirometry); deep inspirations; mucolytic agents.

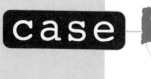

ID/CC A 14-year-old male presents with complaints of **exertional dyspnea, chronic productive cough**, and **occasional hemoptysis.**

HPI He was diagnosed with **cystic fibrosis** at age 4 and has had **recurrent pulmonary infections** requiring frequent hospitalizations.

PE VS: low-grade fever (38°C); tachycardia (HR 110); tachypnea (RR 28). PE: pallor and grade II **clubbing** noted; **coarse crackles** auscultated over both lung fields.

Labs CBC: **normocytic, normochromic anemia**; low hematocrit. Sputum culture reveals *Staphylococcus aureus.* PFTs: decreased FEV_1/FVC suggestive of obstructive pathology.

Imaging XR: chest: increased bronchovascular markings; honeycomb appearance (due to end-on shadows of dilated bronchioles); loss of lung volume (atelectasis). CT (high resolution): chest: **dilated bronchioles with "signet ring" appearance** (due to adjacent branch of pulmonary artery).

Gross Pathology Long, tubelike, irreversibly dilated bronchioles extending to the pleura with loss of lung parenchyma.

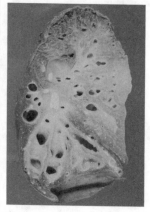

Figure 5-1. The resected upper lobe shows widely dilated bronchi, with thickening of the bronchial walls and collapse and fibrosis of the pulmonary parenchyma.

case  5

Bronchiectasis

Differential

α_1-antitrypsin Deficiency
Asthma
Bronchitis
Chronic Bronchitis
Emphysema
Chronic Obstructive Pulmonary Disease
Pneumonia

Discussion

Dilatation of the bronchial tree leads to infections and to further irreversible dilatation. Underlying causes include **obstruction** due to tumor, foreign bodies, and mucus impaction; **congenital disorders** such as Kartagener's syndrome, Williams-Campbell syndrome, and **cystic fibrosis**; and **infections** due to *Bordetella pertussis,* togavirus, RSV, measles, and *Mycobacterium tuberculosis.* **Complications** include **lung abscesses, metastatic brain abscesses, amyloidosis, and cor pulmonale.**

Treatment

Supportive measures; antibiotics; bronchodilators, expectorants, and **physical therapy** to promote bronchial drainage. Surgery may be indicated for localized or segmental bronchiectasis or when medical therapy fails.

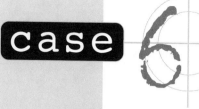

case 6

ID/CC   A **60-year-old male** is referred to an allergist for late-onset **asthma** that has been **unresponsive to bron-chodilators and antibiotics.**

HPI   He has also been having chest pain (ANGINA), fatigue, anorexia, and pain in both calves (CLAUDICATION) on exertion that are of recent onset.

PE   VS: tachypnea; mild fever; **mild hypertension** (BP 150/100) (secondary to renal vascular involvement). PE: marked respiratory distress; widespread **wheezes** bilaterally; numerous **purpuric lesions on feet.**

Labs   CBC: mild anemia; leukocytosis (>10,000/uL); Hct <35%; **eosinophilia (>1000/uL). Elevated BUN and creatinine;** P-ANCA positive; elevated ESR and C-reactive protein. UA: **proteinuria;** presence of **RBCs,** WBCs, and **granular casts.** PFTs: FEV_1/FVC ratio reduced **(obstructive pulmonary disease).** ECG: sinus tachycardia.

Imaging   CXR: **bilateral upper and lower lobe infiltrates** and noncavitating nodules.

Gross Pathology   Lung shows hemorrhagic infarcts secondary to thrombi in affected arteries.

Micro Pathology   Transbronchial lung biopsy shows **granulomatous lesions in vascular and extravascular sites accompanied by intense eosinophilia;** skin biopsy of purpuric lesions shows **vasculitic lesions**—fibrinoid necrosis of media with mixture of inflammatory cells extending along adventitia; occasional aneurysms and secondary thromboses seen; the arterial internal elastic lamina is destroyed and intima and media are thickened.

case 6

Churg-Strauss Syndrome

Differential | Asthma
Eosinophilic Pneumonia
Polyarteritis Nodosa
Wegener Granulomatosis
Microscopic Polyangitis
Goodpasture Syndrome
Pneumonia

Discussion | Churg–Strauss syndrome is an idiopathic systemic **small- and medium-vessel granulomatous vasculitis** (grouped with polyarteritis nodosa [PAN], which does not involve lungs) that is characterized by a triad of late-onset **asthma**, a fluctuating **eosinophilia**, and an **extrapulmonary vasculitis**.

Treatment | **Prednisone** is effective in inducing remission; **cyclophosphamide** or other cytotoxic/immunosuppressive agents when disease is **refractory** to steroids; monitor disease course using **ESR levels**.

■ TABLE 6-1 MAJOR VASCULITIS SYNDROMES

Syndrome	Vessels Involved	Distribution of Vascular Involvement
Polyarteritis nodosa	Medium-sized and small arteries	GI tract, liver, kidney, pancreas, muscles, other sites
Wegener granulomatosis	Small to medium-sized arteries	Upper and lower respiratory tracts; occasionally eye, skin, heart
Microscopic polyangitis (hypersensitivity vasculitis, microscopic polyarteritis)	Venules, capillaries, arterioles	Widespread, but particularly skin
Temporal (cranial) arteritis	Elastic tissue—rich major arteries	Head, including ocular and intracranial vessels; uncommonly systemic
Kawasaki's arteritis	Small to medium-sized arteries	Skin, ocular and oral mucosa, coronary arteries, but may be widespread
Thromboangitis obliterans (Buerger's disease)	Medium-sized and small arteries and veins	Extremities

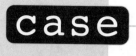

case 7

ID/CC	A 50-year-old white male **smoker** presents with **productive cough, copious sputum,** shortness of breath, and **fever.**
HPI	The patient has a **40-pack-year** smoking history. He has also experienced chronic dyspnea on exertion; chronic **productive cough,** usually **in the mornings,** for several years; and multiple colds each winter.
PE	VS: fever. PE: stocky build with plethora; wheezes.
Labs	CBC: elevated WBC count (14,000); neutrophils predominant; **secondary polycythemia.** *Streptococcus pneumoniae* or *Haemophilus influenzae* on Gram stain of sputum sample. ABGs: decreased Po_2; elevated Pco_2. PFTs: decreased vital capacity; **decreased FEV_1.**
Imaging	CXR: increased bronchovascular markings in lower lung fields.
Gross Pathology	Thick mucous secretion; edema of bronchial mucosa.
Micro Pathology	**Increased size and number of mucous glands,** inflammation; fibrosis; squamous metaplasia.

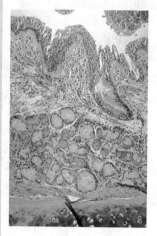

Figure 7-1. The bronchial wall is thickened and shows hyperplasia of the mucus-secreting glands.

13

case  7

Chronic Bronchitis

Differential

Asthma
Bronchiectasis
Chronic Obstructive Pulmonary Disease
Pneumonia
Cystic Fibrosis
Retained Foreign Body

Discussion

Patients present with a history of persistent cough with sputum production for **at least 3 months for at least 2 consecutive years.** They often have **hypercapnia with severe hypoxia,** leading to the term "**Blue Bloaters.**" Histology reveals an **increased Reid Index (>0.5).**

Breakout Point

> Reid index is ratio of thickness of mucus gland to muscular layer in bronchioles

Treatment

Antibiotics; bronchodilators; steroids; home oxygen; **smoking cessation.**

ID/CC	A 55-year-old male complains of progressively increasing **shortness of breath on exertion** for the past few months.
HPI	He also complains of a nonproductive mild cough and has a **40-pack-year smoking history** but has no history of hemoptysis or occupational exposure to inorganic or organic dusts.
PE	VS: moderate tachypnea. PE: moderate respiratory distress; **using accessory muscles of respiration;** fullness of neck veins during expiration; chest **barrel-shaped; percussion note hyperresonant.**
Labs	ABGs: mild hypoxia with respiratory alkalosis. PFTs: increased residual volume; **decreased FEV_1/FVC ratio;** decreased DL_{CO}.
Imaging	CXR (PA view): **hyperlucent** lung fields with a few **bullae;** flattening of diaphragm and elongated tubular heart shadow.
Micro Pathology	Alveolar septa are visibly diminished in number along with increased air spaces.

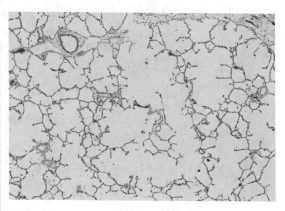

Figure 8-1. Large, irregular air spaces and a markedly reduced number of alveolar walls.

case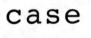

Emphysema

Differential

Asthma

Bronchiectasis

Chronic Bronchitis

Hypersensitivity Pneumonitis

Farmer's Lung

Pneumothorax

Diaphragmatic Paralysis

Discussion

Emphysema is defined as abnormal permanent enlargement of the air spaces distal to the terminal bronchiole accompanied by the destruction of the alveolar walls; emphysema may involve the acinus and the lobule uniformly in a pattern called panacinar, or it may primarily involve the respiratory bronchioles, termed centriacinar. Panacinar emphysema is common in patients with α_1-**antitrypsin deficiency.** Centriacinar emphysema is commonly found in cigarette smokers and is rare in nonsmokers; it is usually more extensive and severe in the upper lobes.

Breakout Point

> Patients with emphysema are often referred to as "Pink Puffers" as they are able to remain well oxygenated as they overventilate as compared to the "Blue Bloaters" with chronic bronchitis.

Treatment

Cessation of smoking, bronchodilators, steroids in resistant cases, antibiotics during acute exacerbations, and home oxygen therapy.

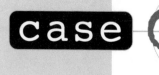

case 9

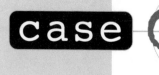

ID/CC   A 58-year-old male complains of **headache**, anxiety, shortness of breath, and increased sleepiness (SOMNOLENCE) while experiencing an **acute exacerbation of COPD**.

HPI   The patient is a **chronic smoker** and also complains of recent **blurring of vision**. He has a history of episodic shortness of breath, mucoid cough, and occasional wheezing (consistent with predominantly **bronchitic COPD**) but no history of neurologic deficit, previous hypertension, or diabetes.

PE   VS: tachycardia; tachypnea; mild systolic hypertension; no fever. PE: anxious and in moderate respiratory distress; using accessory muscles of respiration with prolonged expiration; mild **central cyanosis and pallor; no clubbing;** extremities warm; **flapping tremor of hand** (ASTERIXIS); **bounding pulses** (due to high volume); funduscopy reveals **early papilledema;** chest barrel-shaped with bilateral rhonchi and occasional rales; no focal neurologic deficits.

Labs   ABGs: **hypoxia, hypercapnia, and partially compensated respiratory acidosis.** CBC: polycythemia.

Imaging   CXR (PA view): increased bronchovascular markings (dirty lung fields).

case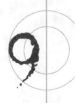

Carbon Dioxide Narcosis

Differential

Asthma

Botulism

Chronic Bronchitis

Hypersensitivity Pneumonitis

Farmer's Lung

Pneumothorax

Diaphragmatic Paralysis

Opioid Abuse

Obesity

Discussion

Dyspnea and headache are the cardinal symptoms of hypercapnia. Hypercapnia also produces a variety of neurologic abnormalities; symptoms include somnolence, blurred vision, restlessness, and anxiety that can progress to tremors, asterixis, delirium, and coma. Supplemental oxygen should be used sparingly to **avoid increasing Pao_2**, which removes the hypoxic respiratory stimulus and leads to respiratory depression.

Treatment

Low-dose continuous oxygen inhalation and, if required, mechanical ventilation to reverse acidosis; broad-spectrum antibiotics, bronchodilators (ipratropium bromide and sympathomimetics), and steroids are used in COPD patients.

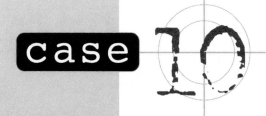

case 10

ID/CC	A 37-year-old **male** in the ICU develops **petechiae, altered sensorium, and marked dyspnea** that prove refractory to oxygen therapy.
HPI	**Twenty-four hours ago,** he was admitted to the hospital with **fractures of the shafts of both femurs, the pelvis, and the right humerus** sustained following a fall from a 20-foot-high ladder.
PE	VS: fever; marked dyspnea. PE: **delirium; central cyanosis;** using accessory muscles of respiration; wheezing heard over both lung fields.
Labs	ABGs: **profound arterial hypoxemia with hypercapnia.** CBC/PBS: thrombocytopenia. **Fat demonstrated in urine and sputum;** normal PT and PTT.
Imaging	CXR: early, normal; later, bilateral perihilar ("BAT-WING") appearance of **pulmonary infiltrates** without cardiomegaly (due to noncardiogenic pulmonary edema). XR, plain: long bone fractures.
Micro Pathology	Obstruction of pulmonary vessels by fat globules; chemical pneumonitis.

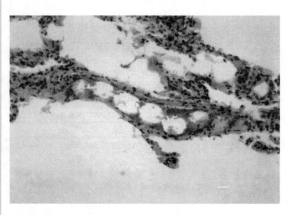

Figure 10-1. Fat globules evident as empty circular spaces within a small pulmonary vessel.

19

case

Fat Embolism

Differential

Pulmonary Embolism

Thrombotic Thrombocytopenic Purpura

Discussion

Fat embolization usually occurs **24 to 72 hours after fractures of the shafts of the long bones.** In most cases the embolization is clinically unapparent; however, in cases of **fat emboli syndrome,** as in this case, the outcome is potentially life threatening. Histologic stains such as Sudan Red can selective stain fat globules with vessels.

Treatment

Intermittent positive pressure ventilation with 100% oxygen, supportive management.

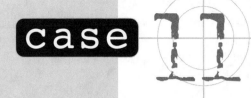

case

ID/CC	A 50-year-old **farmer** presents with severe **shortness of breath** (DYSPNEA) and **fatigue.**
HPI	He also complains of a **dry cough** and **mild fever.** His symptoms are exacerbated when he works in the fields, especially when he comes into contact with **moldy hay.** He does not smoke and drinks alcohol occasionally.
PE	VS: tachycardia; tachypnea; mild fever. PE: moderate respiratory distress; scattered rhonchi and **bilateral fine rales.**
Labs	CBC: leukocytosis with shift to left. Elevated ESR; **serum antibodies against thermophilic *Actinomyces* organisms;** bronchoalveolar lavage shows marked lymphocytosis, primarily suppressor-cytotoxic T cells. PFTs: **restrictive lung disease** pattern.
Imaging	CXR: bilateral **reticulonodular infiltrates with fibrosis.** CT: areas of ground-glass abnormalities with centrilobular peribronchial nodules.
Gross Pathology	Fibrosis with honeycombing.
Micro Pathology	Bronchoscopic lung biopsy reveals interstitial pneumonia with lymphocytes and plasma cells in alveolar walls as well as scattered focal granulomas with foreign body giant cells.

case 11

Hypersensitivity Pneumonitis

Differential

Asbestosis
Coal Worker's Pneumoconiosis
Goodpasture Syndrome
Metastatic Cancer
Mixed Connective Tissue Disease
Idiopathic Pulmonary Fibrosis
Sarcoidosis
Wegener Granulomatosis

Discussion

Hypersensitivity pneumonitis (allergic alveolitis) refers to interstitial lung disease that results from inhalation of organic antigens. Hypersensitivity pneumonitis is believed to have an immunologic basis (e.g., cytotoxic, immune complex, and cell-mediated reactions); **the most common form of hypersensitivity pneumonitis, called farmer's lung, is caused by inhalation of a thermophilic *Actinomyces* organism present in moldy hay and grain.** Other common causes of hypersensitivity pneumonitis include pigeon breeder's disease and bird fancier's disease, in which inhaled serum proteins from pigeons or parakeets induce the syndrome. Humidifier lung disease results from exposure to contaminated forced-air systems.

Treatment

Environmental control to minimize antigen exposure; steroids.

■ TABLE 11-1 CAUSES OF HYPERSENSITIVITY PNEUMONIAS

Disease	Exposure
Farmer's lung	Moldy hay
Bagassosis	Moldy sugar cane fiber
Grain handler's lung	Moldy grain
Humidifier/air-conditioner lung	Contaminated forced-air systems, heated water reservoirs
Bird breeder's lung	Pigeons, parakeets, fowl, rodents
Cheese worker's lung	Cheese mold
Chemical worker's lung	Manufacture of plastics, polyurethane foam, rubber

case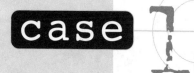

ID/CC   A 65-year-old male complains of progressive shortness of breath on exertion and a chronic **dry cough**.

HPI   The patient has **never smoked** cigarettes and has no history of exposure to occupational dusts or fumes; he has not had a productive cough or hemoptysis.

PE   VS: warm but **cyanosed**; tachycardia (HR 108); tachypnea; BP normal. PE: **clubbing present**; JVP not elevated; heart sounds normal with no additional sounds or murmurs; respiratory examination reveals presence of bilateral **basal fine inspiratory crepitations**.

Labs   ABGs: hypoxemia. PFTs: **decreased DL_{CO}**; desaturation with exercise; proportionately reduced FEV_1 and FVC so that ratio remained unchanged (due to restrictive disease). Bronchoalveolar lavage predominantly neutrophilic; serum calcium and ACE levels low.

Imaging   CXR: reticulonodular shadows in both lower lung fields with occasional areas of "**honeycombing**." CT (high resolution): fibrosis in lower lung lobes suggestive of usual **interstitial pneumonitis pattern of IPF**.

Micro Pathology   Bronchoscopically obtained lung biopsy reveals presence of fibrosis, inflammatory round cell infiltrate, and thickening of the alveolar septa.

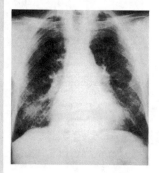

Figure 12-1. The chest radiograph reveals diffuse reticulonodular infiltrates with a predilection for the lung bases.

23

case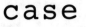

Idiopathic Pulmonary Fibrosis

Differential
Asbestosis
Eosinophilic Granuloma
Hypersensitivity Pneumonitis
Lymphangitis Carcinomatosa
Pneumocystitis Carinii Pneumonia
Pulmonary Edema
Sarcoidosis

Discussion
The main differential diagnoses to consider are lung fibrosis associated with a connective tissue disorder (rule out by history and clinical exam); extrinsic alveolitis due to organic dusts; left-sided heart failure; sarcoidosis (rule out on the basis of absence of any other system involvement, normal calcium and ACE levels, negative Kveim's test, and lack of hilar lymphadenopathy observed on CXR); lymphangitis carcinomatosa (rule out on biopsy and CT); and pneumoconiosis. The onset of idiopathic pulmonary fibrosis is typically in the fifth or sixth decade.

Treatment
Systemic steroids.

case 13

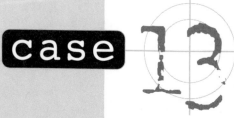

ID/CC A 58-year-old male presents with **shortness of breath** (DYSPNEA), **hoarseness, cough,** and **hemoptysis.**

HPI He has an **80-pack-year smoking history.** Over the past 2 months, he has also had a **significant loss of appetite and weight.**

PE Marked pallor; **cachexia; clubbing;** mild wheezing at rest; chest barrel shaped (emphysematous) and movements diminished on right; **dullness to percussion** over right middle lobe; **no breath sounds** heard over right middle lobe; vocal fremitus reduced in same area.

Labs CBC: **normocytic, normochromic anemia.** Gram and ZN stains of sputum for acid-fast bacilli negative; sputum cytology reveals presence of **malignant cells.**

Imaging CXR/CT: irregular hilar mass on right side, producing an obstruction atelectasis of right middle lobe. Bronchoscopy: right-sided hilar mass obstructing right middle bronchus.

Micro Pathology Biopsy reveals presence of malignant, cellular stratification, **intercellular bridges,** and "**keratin pearls.**"

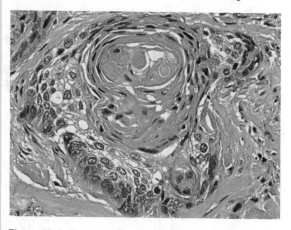

Figure 13-1. Prominent keratinization and keratin pearl formation.

case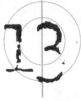

Bronchogenic Carcinoma—Squamous Cell Carcinoma

Differential
Bronchogenic Cyst
Coccioidomycosis
Histoplasmosis
Lung Hematoma
Arteriovenous Malformation
Tuberculosis

Discussion
Lung cancer is the **most preventable cancer.** Owing to the increased incidence of smoking, lung cancer has exceeded breast cancer as the leading cause of cancer death in women. A **Pancoast's tumor** is a lung tumor located at the lung apex in the superior pulmonary sulcus that causes compression of the cervical sympathetic plexus, resulting in **Horner syndrome** as well as scapular pain and ulnar nerve radiculopathy.

Breakout Point

> Breakout Box: Horner syndrome = ptosis, miosis, anhidrosis

Treatment
Surgical resection can be potentially curative in patients with no involvement of surrounding mediastinal structures, contralateral lymph nodes, or distant organs; chemotherapy and/or radiation therapy may be useful in management of unresectable disease.

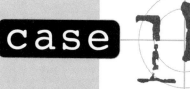

case 14

ID/CC	A 50-year-old **white male uranium miner** presents with **hemoptysis, wheezing, coughing**, dysphagia, **chest pain, shortness of breath**, and **back pain**.
HPI	He has a **40-pack-year smoking history.** He complains of **anorexia, weight loss**, and **fever** for **10 weeks**.
PE	**Icterus**; accessory muscle use, dullness to percussion, and absent breath sounds on the right; distant heart sounds on auscultation; **hepatomegaly**; **edematous right upper extremity**.
Labs	**Elevated LDH; elevated calcium** and alkaline phosphatase; elevated liver enzymes.
Imaging	CXR/CT: **rib destruction, large hilar mass** on the right side, with **loculated pleural effusion.** Bone scan: **increased radiotracer activity** in the **pelvis, spine, ribs,** and **left scapula**. PET scan: **increased uptake in lesion.**
Micro Pathology	Biopsy reveals **neuroendocrine granules** and **Kulchitsky cells** (small, round cells with dark nuclei, scant cytoplasm, fine granular nuclear chromatin, and indistinct nucleoli).

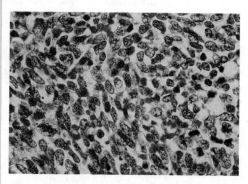

Figure 14-1. This tumor consists of small oval to spindle-shaped cells with scant cytoplasm, finely granular nuclear chromatin, and conspicuous mitoses.

case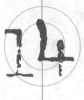

Bronchogenic Carcinoma—Small Cell Carcinoma

Differential

Lymphoma

Non-small Cell Lung Cancer

Bronchogenic Cyst

Leukemia

Neurogenic Tumors

Metastasis from Other Cancers

Discussion

Without treatment, small cell carcinoma is the most aggressive pulmonary tumor, with median survival of only 2 to 4 months from the time of diagnosis. There are 3 types of small cell lung cancer (SCLC)—small cell carcinoma (oat cell carcinoma), mixed small cell/large cell carcinoma, and combined small cell carcinoma. SCLC is one of the most common causes of **SVC syndrome** (gradual, insidious compression/obstruction of the superior vena cava)—**dyspnea and extremity swelling** being the most common symptoms. **Paraneoplastic syndromes** are also common (e.g., SIADH, Eaton-Lambert, subacute sensory neuropathy). This cancer also **frequently metastasizes to the brain, bones, liver, and adrenal glands.**

Treatment

Compared with other cell types of lung cancer, SCLC is usually widely disseminated by the time of diagnosis but is much more responsive to chemotherapy and radiation. Surgery is generally not an option.

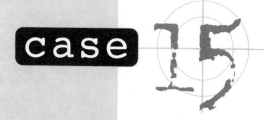

case 15

ID/CC	A 40-year-old, **female nonsmoker** presents with **hemoptysis, mucus-producing cough**, and **wheeze**.
HPI	She complains of recent **weight loss and anorexia;** She works as a **construction worker**, and has been exposed to **second-hand smoke** for many years.
PE	**Clubbing; dullness to percussion** and **decreased breath sounds** on the left; **palpable cervical lymph nodes**.
Labs	**Sputum cytology reveals mucin;** WBCs mildly elevated.
Imaging	CXR/CT: **pleural effusion** in left lung base surrounding a **consolidation**.
Micro Pathology	**Cuboid to columnar cells** that frequently secrete **mucin** identified on **Schiff** staining.

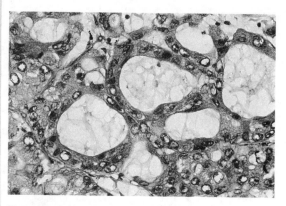

Figure 15-1. Mucinous cuboidal cells.

29

case

Bronchogenic Carcinoma—Adenocarcinoma

Differential

Pneumonia

Metastasis from Other Primary Tumor

Focal Pulmonary Manifestations of Tuberculosis

Lymphoma

Systemic Mycoses

Discussion

Adenocarcinoma is the **most common** type of lung cancer in the United States, usually occurring in a **peripheral** location within the lung and arising from **bronchial mucosal glands.** It may manifest as multifocal tumors in bronchoalveolar form. The WHO classifies adenocarcinomas into four different types: **acinar, papillary, bronchoalveolar, and mucus-secreting.** About 17% of people with adenocarcinoma survive more than 5 years after diagnosis.

Treatment

If the adenocarcinoma is diagnosed in Stage I or II **surgical resection** of the tumor is often an option. Approximately 80% of patients will receive **chemotherapy. Radiation therapy** is also used in treating the adenocarcinoma, often in conjunction with surgical resection.

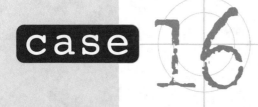

case 16

ID/CC	65 year-old male presents with a cough, **bronchorrhea, shortness of breath, hemoptysis,** and chest pain.
HPI	He is a **nonsmoker,** but has a history of **tuberculosis.** He complains of **unexplained weight loss,** ongoing **fatigue,** and **dyspnea on exertion.**
PE	**Cachexia; dullness to percussion** and **absent breath sounds** on the right.
Labs	**WBC count: within normal limits.**
Imaging	CXR/CT scan: dense parenchymal **consolidation** in the right lower lobe with air bronchograms, **enhancing pulmonary vessels** seen within the consolidated lung. Multiple **smaller nodular densities** seen in the contralateral lung.
Micro Pathology	Three cell types—**Clara cells, type II pneumocytes,** and **mucin producing cells.** Mucin producing cells stain **PAS-D positive.** Malignant cells line the alveoli called "**tomb stone**" cells.

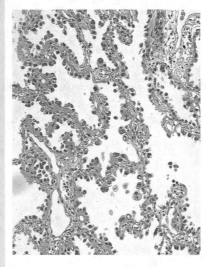

Figure 16-1. Intra-alveolar growth of tumor cells.

31

case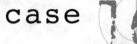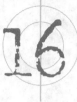

Bronchogenic Carcinoma—Bronchoalveolar Carcinoma

Differential

Lymphoma
Sarcoidosis
Lipoid Pneumonia
Tuberculosis
Alveolar Proteinosis

Discussion

Most patients who present with bronchoalveolar carcinoma have a history of **scarred lung** (i.e., from tuberculosis, scleroderma, fibrosis), and **one-third** of the patients are **nonsmokers.** Sixty percent of the patients were identified by routine chest x-rays and were asymptomatic on presentation. Bronchoalveolar carcinoma, a **subtype of large cell lung cancer,** is more inclined to stay within the lung and is less likely to spread to other organs. The tumor tends to be **peripherally** based. In multifocal tumors, the lung architecture remains preserved—hemorrhage, necrosis, and cavitation are almost always absent. Bronchoalveolar carcinoma is **often confused with pneumonia** or other inflammatory conditions in the lung, so if a patient fails antibiotic therapy this diagnosis should be entertained.

Treatment

The tumor is usually treated with **surgery, chemotherapy,** and **radiation therapy.** Massive bronchorrea responds best to radiation therapy.

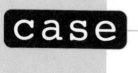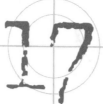

ID/CC	A 50-year-old, male **nonsmoker** presents to his physician with complaints of a productive cough and wheeze.
HPI	The patient has had multiple recent hospitalizations with pneumonia. He does admit to occasional **asthma-like symptoms** and several episodes of coughing up **blood tinged sputum**.
PE	Vital signs stable, lung exam demonstrates **end expiratory wheeze** with a prolonged **expiratory wheeze**. His extremities display no clubbing.
Labs	CBC within normal limits; PFT within normal limits.
Imaging	CXR demonstrates partial collapse of the left lower lobe. CT scan of the chest demonstrates a soft tissue density within the left main bronchus. Bronchoscopy demonstrates a fleshy polypoid mass with some fresh bleeding protruding into the left main bronchus.
Gross Pathology	3-cm **polypoid mass protruding into the bronchial lumen** with intact overlaying mucosa.
Micro Pathology	Kulchitsky cell differentiation. Cells stain positive for amine precursor uptake and decarboxylation (**APUD**) markers.

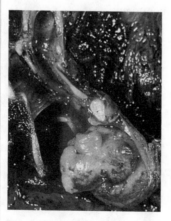

Figure 17-1. Endobronchial polypoid lesion.

case 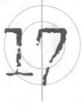 17

Bronchial Carcinoid

Differential

Pulmonary Aspergillosis

Small Cell Lung Cancer

Tuberculosis

Arteriovenous Malformation

Pulmonary Metastasis

Non-Hodgkin Lymphoma

Discussion

Although rare tumors, bronchial carcinoids represent a distinct class of neuroendocrine tumors. They are distinctly different from the neuroendocrine cells scene in small cell lung cancer. Like other APUD cells they have the capability of producing serotonin, ACTH, norepinephrine, ADH, and Bradykinen. However, they cause paraneoplastic syndromes far less common than small cell carcinomas. They tend to be low-**grade malignancies** that cause local invasion and tend to recur. They are often highly vascular and often bleed, causing hemoptysis.

Treatment

The tumors are generally **resistant to most forms of chemotherapy** and therefore are generally surgically resected, and in select cases can be conservatively monitored.

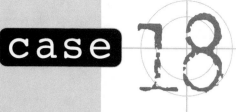

case 18

PULMONOLOGY

ID/CC A 67-year-old male is referred to a clinic for evaluation of **pleuritic pain, weight loss,** gradually progressive **dyspnea,** and a **nonproductive cough** of a few months' duration.

HPI He worked in a **shipyard** for 20 years before retiring, an occupation that involved **asbestos exposure.**

PE VS: normal. PS: **clubbing of fingers;** mild cyanosis; **reduced chest expansion; dull percussion, reduced breath sounds,** and egophony in right side (due to pleural effusion).

Labs CBC/PBS: polycythemia; **marked eosinophilia.** PFTs: **restrictive pattern** observed (decreased vital capacity and decreased total lung capacity with normal FEV_1/FVC ratio). Reduced diffusion capacity; pleural effusion bloody and shows acidic pH (<7.3).

Imaging CXR: right-sided pleural effusion; diffuse bilateral **interstitial fibrosis; parietal pleural calcifications.** CT: highly irregular pleural-based masses; hemorrhagic effusion.

Gross Pathology Thick, **fibrous pleural plaques with calcification.**

Micro Pathology Epithelioid pattern of pleural malignant sarcomatous transformation with cellular atypia and high mitotic index.

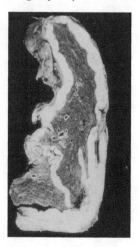

Figure 18-1. Pleural malignant mesothelioma. The lung is encased by a dense pleural tumor, which extends along the interlobar fissures but does not involve the underlying lung parenchyma.

35

case

Malignant Mesothelioma

Differential
Nonsmall Cell Carcinoma
Small Cell Carcinoma
Congestive Heart Failure
Metastatic Cancer

Discussion
Occupational exposure to asbestos is found in 80% of cases of malignant mesothelioma; it produces **lung fibrosis** with a **restrictive pattern.** Asbestos and tobacco exposure synergistically increase the risk of lung adenocarcinoma.

Treatment
Surgery, chemotherapy, radiation therapy, and multi-modality treatments may be employed; poor prognosis.

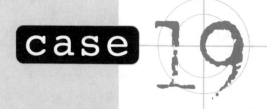

ID/CC	A 37-year-old female comes to the emergency room complaining of **pleuritic pain** on the right side of her chest and **dyspnea** together with fever and a productive cough.
HPI	There is no hemoptysis. The pain is typically **sharp and stabbing,** and it arises when she takes a deep breath (PLEURISY).
PE	**Decreased chest movement during inhalation** on right side; **dullness** on percussion of right lung base; **reduced or absent breath sounds** over right lung base; bronchial breath sounds auscultated on right side; friction rub; location of **dullness moves with respiration; decreased tactile fremitus** over right lung.
Labs	CBC: elevated WBC count with predominance of neutrophils. Grampositive diplococci on sputum smear and culture; **elevated protein, decreased glucose, and many neutrophils in pleural exudate.**
Imaging	CXR: lateral decubitus: **layering of fluid.**

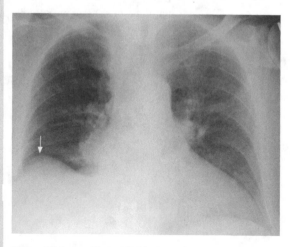

Figure 19-1. Layering of fluid

37

case

Pleural Effusion

Differential
Nonsmall Cell Carcinoma
Small Cell Carcinoma
Congestive Heart Failure
Metastatic Cancer

Discussion
Pleural effusions may be due to infection (viral, bacterial, mycobacterial, fungal); other causes are malignancies, congestive heart failure, cirrhosis, nephrotic syndrome, trauma, pancreatitis, collagen diseases, and drug reactions. Effusions may be **transudative** (<3 g/dL of protein) or **exudative** (>3 g/dL of protein). Elevated pleural fluid LDH levels may be suggestive of malignancy. **Transudative pleural effusions** are commonly caused by congestive heart failure, cirrhosis, and nephrotic syndrome, whereas **exudative pleural effusions** are caused by TB, infections, malignancy, pancreatitis, pulmonary embolus, and chylothorax (milky pleural fluid).

Treatment
Antibiotics and needle drainage of effusion (THORACENTESIS); sometimes obliteration of pleural space with talc or other compounds (pleuradysis).

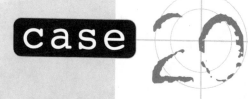

ID/CC A 25-year-old white **male** complains of **sudden pleuritic chest pain** and **shortness of breath** that **awakens him at night.**

HPI He **smokes** one pack of cigarettes a day and states that his paternal **uncle once had a similar episode.**

PE **Tall, thin** patient; diaphoretic and feels weak; left chest expands poorly on inspiration; trachea and apex beat displaced to right; left side **hyperresonant** to percussion; **decreased breath sounds; decreased tactile fremitus.**

Labs ABGs: decreased P_{O_2}; elevated P_{CO_2}.

Imaging CXR: partial collapse of left lung with no lung markings except **thin line parallel to chest wall; costophrenic sulcus abnormally radiolucent** ("DEEP SULCUS" SIGN) in supine film.

Gross Pathology Types: traumatic, spontaneous, tension, open; common causes: surgical puncture, rupture of emphysematous bullae, positive pressure mechanical ventilation, bronchopleural fistula.

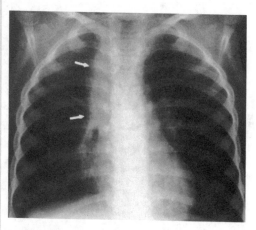

Figure 20-1. Collapse of one portion of the right upper lobe.

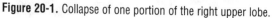

case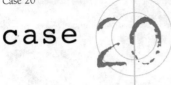

Spontaneous Pneumothorax

Differential
Asthma
Acute Coronary Syndrome
Pulmonary Edema
Costochondritis
Rib Fracture
Tension Pneumothorax
Pulmonary Embolism
Myocarditis
Esophageal Perforation
Pneumonia

Discussion
The usual cause of spontaneous pneumothorax is rupture of a **subpleural bleb**. It is associated with **bullous emphysema** and infectious agents such as tuberculosis.

Treatment
Pneumothorax evacuation via pleural catheter (CHEST TUBE).

case

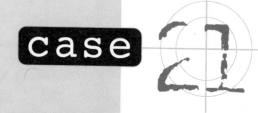

ID/CC	A 40-year-old male is brought to the ER with complaints of **sudden-onset, severe, right-sided chest pain followed by severe difficulty breathing.**
HPI	He is a chronic smoker and has predominantly **emphysematous COPD.**
PE	VS: severe tachycardia; tachypnea; hypotension; no fever. PE: **cyanosis; trachea shifted** to left; chest exam reveals **hyperresonant percussion note on right, diminished breath sounds,** and **decreased tactile fremitus.**
Labs	ABGs: hypoxemia; respiratory alkalosis. ECG: normal.
Imaging	CXR (after patient stabilizes): **shifting of mediastinum toward left.** Flattened left hemidiaphragm.

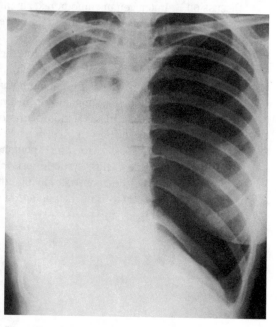

Figure 21-1. Dramatic shift of the left hemithorax.

41

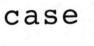

case 21

Tension Pneumothorax

Differential
Asthma
Acute Coronary Syndrome
Aortic Dissection
Rib Fracture
Spontaneous Pneumothorax
Esophageal Perforation
Cardiac Tamponade

Treatment
Immediate life-saving treatment consists of inserting a wide-bore IV cannula in the second intercostal space on the affected side to decompress the pleural cavity if a chest drain is not immediately available; the wide-bore needle can then be replaced by a chest drain connected to an underwater seal.

Discussion
In tension pneumothorax, air enters the pleural space during inspiration and is prevented from escaping during expiration (because an airway or tissue flap acts as a one-way valve); there is a progressive increase in pleural air, which is under pressure (i.e., tension). Tension pneumothorax can occur in cases of idiopathic spontaneous pneumothorax; it is a more common manifestation of the barotrauma that may occur during positive pressure mechanical ventilation. Risk factors for spontaneous pneumothorax include COPD, cystic fibrosis, asthma, and tuberculosis. To demonstrate pneumothorax at autopsy, the chest cavity is opened under water, letting air bubbles escape.

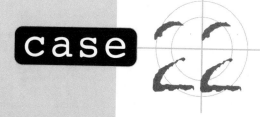

case 22

ID/CC	A **34-year-old**, white, obese **female** complains of **shortness of breath**, dizziness, and near-fainting spells.
HPI	She has been taking **prescription medication** for approximately 6 months in order to **lose weight**.
PE	Obesity; mild cyanosis; **large "a" wave** in jugular venous pressure; parasternal heave; **loud S2**; narrow splitting of S2; rales on both bases; hepatomegaly.
Labs	CBC: **polycythemia**. ECG: **right-axis deviation; right ventricle and right atrial hypertrophy**. ABGs: hypoxemia.
Imaging	CXR: enlarged right ventricle; enlarged main pulmonary artery with peripheral pruning.
Gross Pathology	Enlarged right ventricle with myocardial fiber hypertrophy; atherosclerosis of pulmonary artery; narrowing of arterioles.
Micro Pathology	Atheromas in main elastic arteries. Thickening of the media and intima in medium-size muscular arteries, causing near-obliteration of the lumen.

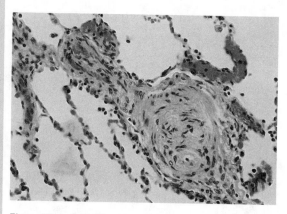

Figure 22-1. A small pulmonary artery is virtually occluded by concentric intimal fibrosis.

43

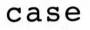

case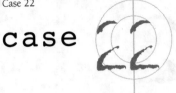

Primary Pulmonary Hypertension

Differential

Sleep Apnea
Dilated Cardiomyopathy
Hypothyroidism
Mitral Stenosis
Mixed Connective Tissue Disease
Secondary Pulmonary Hypertension
Scleroderma

Discussion

Primary pulmonary hypertension is a pathologic increase in pulmonary artery pressure; if long-standing, it causes fatal right heart failure. It may be primary (idiopathic) or secondary to intrinsic pulmonary disease.

Treatment

Calcium channel blockers; prostacyclin; endothelin receptor antagonists; inhaled nitric oxide; heart-lung transplantation can be considered.

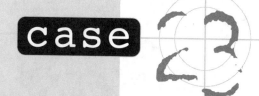

case 23

ID/CC	A 60-year-old female who had undergone right **total hip replacement** presents on the sixth postoperative day with central **chest pain** and **acute-onset dyspnea**.
HPI	She has been **immobile** since the surgery.
PE	VS: low-grade fever; tachycardia; **tachypnea; hypotension.** PE: central cyanosis; **elevated JVP; right ventricular gallop rhythm with widely split S2.**
Labs	ABGs: **hypoxia and hypercapnia** (type 2 respiratory failure). ECG: **S1Q3T3** pattern and sinus **tachycardia.** Positive D-dimer test.
Imaging	CXR: right lower lobe atelectasis. V/Q: three areas of ventilation-perfusion mismatch in right lung. Spiral CT: chest: filling defect in right main pulmonary artery suggestive of an occlusive embolus. Angio, pulmonary: confirmatory; not required if V/Q scan is high probability. US: Doppler: **clot in right common femoral vein.**
Gross Pathology	Large thrombus seen in pulmonary artery.
Micro Pathology	Large occlusive thrombus seen in pulmonary artery with variable degree of recanalization.

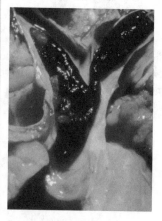

Figure 23-1. The main pulmonary artery and its bifurcation have been opened to reveal a large thrombus.

case

Pulmonary Embolism

Differential | Anemia
Angina
Cardiogenic Shock
Aortic Stenosis
Myocardial Infarction
Pneuomothorax
Septic Shock
Toxic Shock Syndrome

Discussion | Pulmonary emboli most commonly originate from proximal deep venous thrombosis. Pulmonary angiography is the gold standard in the diagnosis of pulmonary embolism, but obtain a V/Q scan initially if clinically suspected. **Virchow's triad** outlines the risk factors for thrombus formation. Large emboli may cause cardiovascular collapse and sudden death.

Breakout Point |

> Virchow's triad = stasis (immobilization), endothelial damage, and hypercoagulable state (i.e., malignancy, pregnancy, severe burn)

Treatment | Supportive; thrombolytic therapy; consider embolectomy; heparin, Coumadin, and low-molecular-weight heparin (enoxaparin) instituted for prophylaxis (monitor INR).

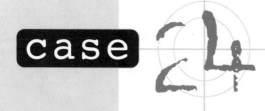

case 24

ID/CC A **28-year-old black female** complains of **fever, dyspnea, arthralgia, and erythematous, tender nodules** on both legs.

HPI She has no history of foreign travel or contact with a tubercular patient.

PE VS: fever. PE: tender, **erythematous nodules over extensor aspects of both legs** (ERYTHEMA NODOSUM); arthralgias of both knees; splenomegaly.

Labs CBC: **lymphopenia; eosinophilia.** Lytes: **elevated serum calcium; hypercalciuria.** ACE levels elevated; blood cultures negative; **Mantoux test negative;** fungal serology negative. PFTs: **evidence of restrictive changes.** Transbronchial lung biopsy ordered.

Imaging XR: **bilateral hilar lymphadenopathy** and right paratrachealadenopathy; **interstitial infiltrates;** no pleural effusion.

Micro Pathology Lymph node biopsy reveals **noncaseating granulomas** with fibrotic acellular core surrounded by lymphocytes, epithelioid cells, and Langerhan's giant cells.

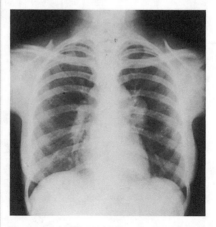

Figure 24-1. Bilateral hilar adenopathy and paratracheal adenopathy with normal lung fields.

case

Sarcoidosis

Differential	Cat-scratch Disease
	Small Cell Lung Cancer
	Non-small Cell Lung Cancer
	Non-Hodgkin Lymphoma
	Hodgkin Lymphoma
	Tuberculosis
	Berylliosis

Discussion In the United States, the incidence of sarcoidosis is highest in black women, with onset between 20 and 40 years of age. The disease may be asymptomatic; however, symptoms may be constitutional and may involve many different organ systems, including the lungs, lymph nodes, skin, eye, upper respiratory tract, reticuloendothelial system, liver, kidneys, nervous system, and heart. Approximately 60% to 70% of sarcoidosis patients recover with few or no residual symptoms.

Treatment **Corticosteroids.**

case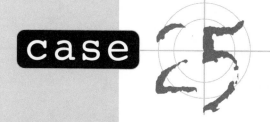

ID/CC	A 56-year-old male presents with progressively increasing **dyspnea** and **dry cough** of several years' duration.
HPI	He is a nonsmoker, but his occupational history includes **mining and quarrying**.
PE	No clubbing, cyanosis, or lymphadenopathy; **reduced chest expansion** on inspiration; **dry inspiratory crackles** auscultated in upper lobes of both lungs.
Labs	PFTs: combined **obstructive and restrictive pattern** of functional impairment. Bronchoscopically-guided lung biopsy establishes diagnosis; negative Mantoux test; sputum cytology and staining for acid-fast bacilli negative.
Imaging	CXR, PA: rounded small opacities in upper lobes with retraction and **hilar lymphadenopathy**; "eggshell" calcification of lymph nodes.
Micro Pathology	Hyalinized whorls of collagen with little or no inflammation.

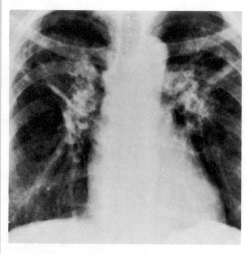

Figure 25-1. Characteristic eggshell lymph node calcifications associated with bilateral perihilar masses.

case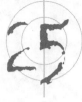

Silicosis

Differential | Asbestosis
Myobacterium Infection
Tuberculosis
Coal Worker's Lung
Sarcoidosis

Discussion | There is an **increased incidence of tuberculosis** in silicosis patients. Silicosis, coal worker's pneumoconiosis, and asbestosis are all forms of pneumoconiosis, or "dust diseases." They ultimately lead to restrictive lung disease that varies in severity from mild to disabling.

Treatment | Supportive; avoidance of further exposure.

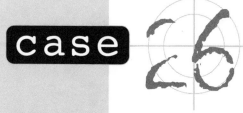

case 26

ID/CC	A 45-year-old Hispanic female is brought to the gynecologist for an evaluation of a **gross difference in the size of her breasts** of recent origin.
HPI	Her medical history is unremarkable. Despite the recent increase in the size of her right breast, she **does not feel any pain and feels only a sensation of fullness.**
PE	**Very large mass** with **firm, "wooden-log" consistency** involving almost all of right breast, making it twice the size of opposite breast; **mobile mass;** appears **well circumscribed; collateral bluish veins seen on skin** along with striae; no peau d'orange appearance; no nipple retraction, axillary lymphadenopathy, or hepatomegaly; opposite breast normal.
Imaging	US: large, smooth multilobulated mass.
Gross Pathology	Large tumor with numerous **cystic spaces on cut section of stroma, producing recesses and longitudinal openings** and causing a leaflike appearance.
Micro Pathology	Abundance of normal-looking ducts, acini, and stroma with no signs of cellular atypia and low mitotic index.

GYNECOLOGY

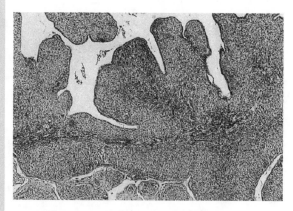

Figure 26-1. Cellular stroma with high mitotic rate and epithelial lined leaf-like architecture.

case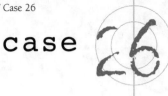

Cystosarcoma Phyllodes

Differential

Angiosarcoma

Breast Carcinoma

Fibroadenoma

Breast Sarcoma

Gynecomastia

Discussion

A less common benign tumor of breast that is also known as giant fibroadenoma, cystosarcoma phyllodes is a **bulky tumor** that, although usually benign histologically, **may recur** following excision and sometimes undergoes malignant degeneration (5% to 10%). It can occur at any age and is more common in African American females. It is thought to be due, in part, to localized hypersensitivity to gonadal hormones. It **rarely metastasizes** to lymph nodes or distant sites.

Treatment

Wide local excision with a rim of normal breast tissue or mastectomy.

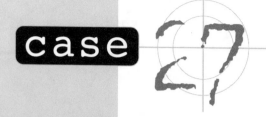
ID/CC A 27-year-old **woman** who is **actively training** for a marathon notes a **painful lump** in the upper outer quadrant of her right breast of 2 days' duration.

HPI She has no history of fever and no known family history of breast cancer.

PE **Retraction of overlying skin** in upper outer quadrant of right breast; **indurated lesion** the size of a lemon in same area; axillary lymph nodes not palpable.

Imaging Mammo: **irregular mass** with **focal areas** of **eggshell calcification.** US: solid, ill-defined mass with altered surrounding architecture.

Gross Pathology Yellowish, fatty fluid on aspiration.

Micro Pathology Excisional biopsy shows localized area of **granulation tissue** within which are numerous lipid-laden macrophages subjacent to necrotic fat cells.

GYNECOLOGY

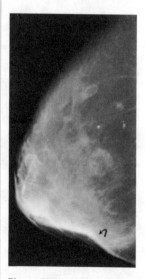

Figure 27-1. Mammogram obtained 6 months after blunt trauma to the breast with skin thickening and retraction (arrow) and multiple egg shell calcifications.

case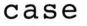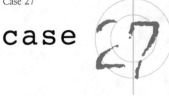

Fat Necrosis of the Breast

Differential
Mastitis
Breast Carcinoma
Fibroadenoma
Breast Sarcoma

Discussion
Fat necrosis of the breast is a unilateral localized process associated with **trauma**, breast biopsy, reduction mammoplasty, and radiation. It is easily confused with cancer due to induration, fibrosis, dystrophic calcification, and retraction of overlying skin; the key distinction is the **presence of pain.** However, biopsy is necessary for definitive diagnosis. The calcification result from **saponification** of fat with the formation of calcium salts that form the areas of calcification.

Treatment
No other active management required.

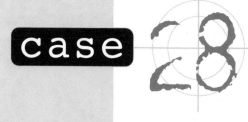

case 28

ID/CC A 32-year-old woman presents with **painful bilateral breast masses**.

HPI The **pain is cyclic** in nature and **increases in her premenstrual phase**, at which time the **masses enlarge rapidly and then shrink**. She feels that both breasts are nodular and is concerned that she may have cancer.

PE Mildly tender mass palpable in upper and outer quadrant of right and left breast; both **breasts nodular with multiple thickened areas**; no changes in overlying skin or nipple noted; no axillary lymphadenopathy found.

Labs Aspiration from breast mass reveals nonbloody fluid; **mass disappears completely after aspiration**.

Imaging Mammo: nodularity and benign calcifications, no malignant features.

Gross Pathology Cysts of various sizes ranging from microscopic to several millimeters surrounded by dense fibrotic tissue; contains clear or brown fluid.

Micro Pathology Proliferation of acini in lobules (SCLEROSING ADENOSIS).

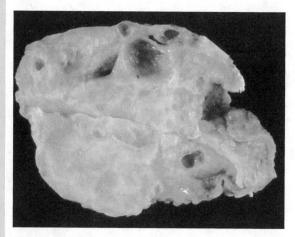

Figure 28-1. Surgical specimen: Cysts of various sizes are dispersed in dense, fibrous connective tissue.

55

case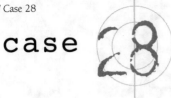

Fibrocystic Disease of the Breast

Differential

Breast Abscess

Fat Necrosis

Fibroadenoma

Breast Carcinoma

Discussion

Fibrocystic disease of the breast is common in women between the ages of 35 and 55 and carries an increased risk of invasive breast cancer in patients with epithelial hyperplasia and atypia. Fibrocystic changes may result from hormone imbalances with either an excess of estrogen or a deficiency of progesterone.

Treatment

Reassurance and symptomatic management.

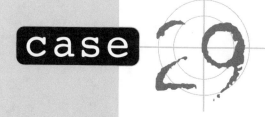

case 29

ID/CC	A 59-year-old white female comes to her family doctor because of a presumed "infection" in her right **breast**; she complains of **pain and swelling**.
HPI	Her history is unremarkable.
PE	VS: **no fever** or other systemic sign of infection. PE: right breast warm, **rock-hard, and swollen with no areas of fluctuation; one-third of breast erythematous** with shiny overlying skin having **peau d'orange** appearance; **painful** to touch and pressure; several axillary **lymph nodes enlarged** and **firm**; some **coalescent**.
Labs	Routine lab work normal.
Micro Pathology	Large spheroidal cells and fine stroma infiltrated by lymphocytes on breast skin biopsy; lymphatic vessels occluded by tumor cells; immunostaining positive for overexpression of HER2/neu.

GYNECOLOGY

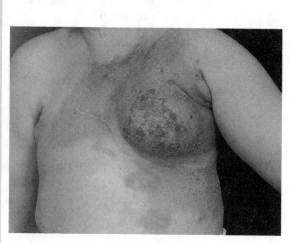

Figure 29-1. Patient on presentation.

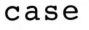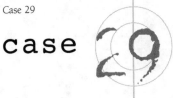

case 29

Inflammatory Carcinoma of the Breast

Differential

Cellulitis

Mastitis

Duct Ectasia

Breast Abscess

Lymphoma

Dermatitis

Discussion

Inflammatory carcinoma of the breast is defined as breast cancer with angiolymphatic spread; it is characterized by a malignant course with early and widespread metastases. Perform skin biopsy in patients diagnosed with breast infection who do not respond promptly to antibiotic treatment. Overexpression of Her2/neu is normally associated with poor prognosis. However, in the age of targeted therapies such a Trastuzumab, such patients can be treated with immunotherapy.

Treatment

Combined-modality treatment with initial induction chemotherapy followed by surgery and/or radiation. Patients overexpressing Her2/neu are treated with **Trastuzumab.**

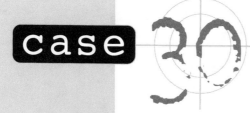

case 30

ID/CC A **35-year-old** female rushes to the emergency room and waits to see a doctor because she is concerned about a **bloody nipple discharge** that she discovered this morning.

HPI She exercises, is very health conscious, and always has safe sex.

PE Palpation around left nipple reveals **blood coming from one of the duct openings** and a **small, soft lump** beneath areola; no breast masses or axillary lymphadenopathy.

Imaging Mammo: negative. Ductography: dilated duct with intraluminal filling defect.

Gross Pathology Epithelial papillary growth with fibrotic components, characteristically located **within a lactiferous duct.**

Micro Pathology No cellular atypia or anaplastic changes on specimen of bloody discharge; only blood intermixed with foamy macrophages and benign ductal epithelium with fibrovascular core.

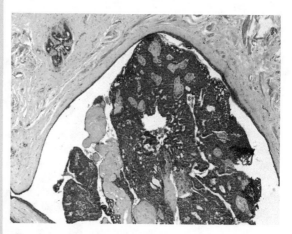

Figure 30-1. A benign papillary growth occupies a subareolar duct.

59

case

Intraductal Papilloma

Differential | Nipple Adenoma
Adenomyoepithelioma
Infiltrating Ductal Papilloma

Discussion | Papilloma of the breast is a benign proliferation of ductal epithelial tissue and is the most common cause of serous/sanguineous discharge.

Treatment | Surgical resection of lactiferous duct (MICRODOCHEC-TOMY) followed by histologic examination to rule out carcinoma.

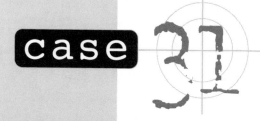

ID/CC A 46-year-old **woman** presents with a palpable mass in the left breast.

HPI The patient has been admitted to the hospital to obtain an excisional biopsy and for planning further management. The **patient's older sister recently died of metastatic breast cancer.**

PE Left breast mass on palpation; nipples normally located without evidence of retraction; no evidence of axillary lymphadenopathy or hepatomegaly.

Imaging Mammo: frequently normal or an asymmetric density without definable margins.

Gross Pathology Firm, white, irregularly shaped 3-cm mass was removed from each breast.

Micro Pathology Histologic sections reveal terminal lobules distended by intermediate-sized cells with scant mitotic activity; neoplastic cells infiltrate the stroma with individual neoplastic cells in a single file (INDIAN FILE PATTERN) that surrounds the terminal lobule in a target-appearing fashion.

GYNECOLOGY

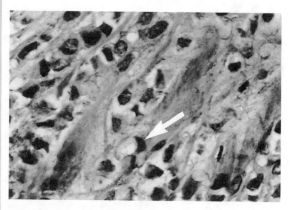

Figure 31-1. Single-file arrangement of cells with pleomorphic nuclei within a fibrous stroma; presence of a signet ring cell.

case

Lobular Carcinoma of the Breast

Differential

Lobular Carcinoma in Situ (LCIS)

Mucinous Carcinoma of the Breast

Lymphoma

Infiltrating Ductal Carcinoma of the Breast

Discussion

Infiltrating lobular carcinoma is the most common malignancy of the terminal lobule. It accounts for 10% to 13% of all breast cancers.

Treatment

Modified radical mastectomy with sentinel lymph node biopsy; radiotherapy and adjuvant chemotherapy. Frequent mammographic surveillance is needed owing to the **high incidence of a second primary in the same or opposite breast.**

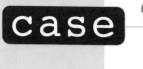
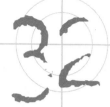

case 32

ID/CC   A 68-year-old white woman visits her dermatologist because of a long-standing **itching, painless, scaling, and oozing erythematous rash** over her right **nipple**.

HPI   Her **first menstrual period** started at **age 9,** and she has **never** been married nor **had children**; her **menopause started at age 56.**

PE   **Nipple** on right breast **retracted** and appears **eczematous** with **redness,** some edema, and **desquamation; oozing** of yellowish exudate; painless left axillary **lymphadenopathy;** no hepatomegaly or lumps in opposite breast.

Gross Pathology   Ductal carcinoma with extension to overlying skin.

Micro Pathology   Characteristic cells are scattered in the epidermis and are mucin positive and have large nuclei and abundant, pale-staining cytoplasm (PAGET'S CELLS); immunohistochemistry for determining estrogen/progesterone receptor status.

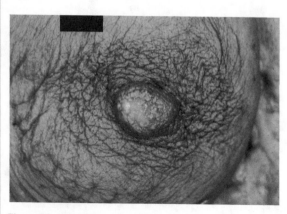

Figure 32-1. Erosion and crusting of the nipple.

63

case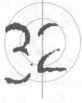

Paget's Disease of the Breast

Differential

Contact Dermatitis

Drug Eruption

Localized Amyloidosis

Malignant Melanoma

Toker Cell Hyperplasia

Discussion

Paget's carcinoma is a scaly skin lesion in the **areola and nipple** arising from **ductal adenocarcinoma** within subareolar excretory ducts and progressing outward.

Breakout Point

> Although Paget's disease of the breast is almost always associated with underlying carcinoma, Paget's disease of the vulva is not.

Treatment

Modified radical mastectomy with axillary lymph node dissection; adjuvant tamoxifen therapy when associated ductal carcinoma is estrogen and progesterone receptor positive.

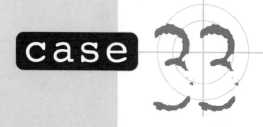

case 33

ID/CC	A **52-year-old** unmarried white **nulliparous female** smoker with **early menarche** presents with a **painless lump** in her right breast.
HPI	The patient has a **history of atypical hyperplasia** of the right breast. Her **mother died of breast cancer** at 46 years of age.
PE	A 3-cm, **fixed, hard, and nontender mass** in **upper outer quadrant** of right breast; **retraction of overlying skin and nipple;** no nipple discharge; **palpable axillary lymph nodes** on right side.
Labs	Routine lab work normal; normal alkaline phosphatase (no bone metastases).
Imaging	Mammo: **spiculated mass with architectural distortion and multiple clustered pleomorphic microcalcifications;** skin thickening and retraction. CXR: no evidence of metastasis.
Gross Pathology	Hard, irregular whitish mass with granules of calcification and focal yellow areas of necrosis.
Micro Pathology	FNA: large pleomorphic cells arranged in glands, cords, nests, and sheets in dense fibrous stroma; cells **estrogen and progesterone receptor negative** by flow cytometry.

GYNECOLOGY

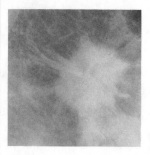

Figure 33-1. Magnified view of a mammogram showing an ill-defined, irregular, spiculated mass.

case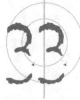

Infiltrating Ductal Carcinoma

Differential

Infiltrating Lobular Carcinoma
Sclerosing Adenosis
Fibrocystic Change
Fibroadenoma
Ductal Carcinoma in Situ

Discussion

Infiltrating ductal breast carcinoma is the **most common type of breast cancer.** This tumor histology is often associated with profound **fibrosis with induration** in stroma (DESMOPLASTIC REACTION). Approximately one in nine women in the United States will develop breast cancer. Risk factors include **family history, early menarche, late menopause, obesity, exogenous estrogens, atypical hyperplasia of breast, and breast cancer in the opposite breast.**

Treatment

Surgery; adjuvant chemotherapy; radiation therapy for selected cases; hormonal agents (e.g., tamoxifen) depending on estrogen and progesterone receptor status; Traztuzamab therapy if the patient's tumors are Her2 positive; rehabilitative measures such as breast reconstruction surgery.

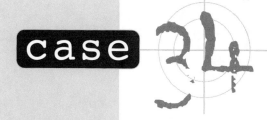

ID/CC   A **25-year-old** black female visits her family doctor for a **painless right breast lump** that she discovered on self-examination; she is otherwise asymptomatic.

HPI   Her medical history is unremarkable.

PE   **Small, encapsulated, well-defined, rubbery, freely movable** 3-cm mass in right lower quadrant of right breast; no overlying skin changes; no nipple retraction; no lymphadenopathy; other breast normal.

Labs   All routine lab work normal.

Imaging   Mammo: oval low-density lesion with smooth margins; **"popcorn calcifications"** seen with degeneration. US: homogeneous, well-circumscribed, hypoechoic mass with visible echogenic capsule.

Gross Pathology   Solid mass; no areas of necrosis or hemorrhage (central myxoid degeneration in older patients).

Micro Pathology   Glandular structures with ductal and stromal proliferation with no cellular atypia.

GYNECOLOGY

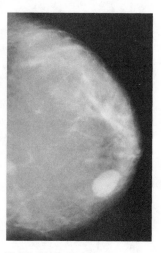

Figure 34-1. Smooth, rounded mass with clearly delineated margins.

case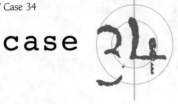

Fibroadenoma

Differential

Phyllodes Tumor
Fibrocystic Change of the Breast
Hematoma
Breast Carcinoma

Treatment

Surgical excision.

Discussion

Fibroadenoma is the **most common benign breast tumor in young women;** given its responsiveness to gonadal steroids, it sometimes enlarges during pregnancy or normal menstrual cycles. It most often occurs in the inner quadrants and is freely moveable. They are usually solitary lesions, which can be very large (>500 g) in the case of giant fibroadenomas. The cells of this benign neoplasm arise from the epithelial and stroma elements of the terminal duct lobular unit.

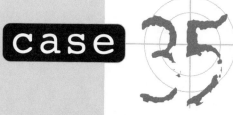

ID/CC A 22-year-old **female** presents with an **abnormal cervical Pap smear.**

HPI She has no history of irregular menstrual bleeding, postcoital bleeding, intermenstrual bleeding, or vaginal discharge. She delivered her **first baby at the age of 18** and has had **multiple sexual partners.**

Imaging Colposcopy reveals a suspicious area from which a biopsy is taken.

Micro Pathology Biopsy shows loss of normal orientation of squamous cells; atypical cells seen with wrinkled nuclei and perinuclear halos involving full thickness of squamous epithelium; **basement membrane intact.**

GYNECOLOGY

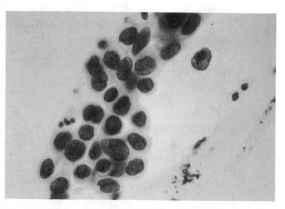

Figure 35-1. Pap smear showing small cells with hyperchromatic nuclei irregular nuclear contours and scant cytoplasm.

case

Cervical Carcinoma in Situ

Differential

Endocervical Polyp

Cervical Leiomyoma

Complex Nabothian Cyst

Endometrial Carcinoma

Cervicitis

Discussion

Cervical dysplasia is a precursor of cervical squamous cell carcinoma; it is associated with **infection with human papillomavirus (HPV) types 16, 18, and 31.** The oncoprotein E6 of HPV inactivates the cellular tumor suppressor gene p53, whereas the viral E7 inhibits the tumor suppressor gene Rb (retinoblastoma). This results in derangement of the cell cycle leading to cancer. Cervical cancer screenings with Pap smears have dramatically decreased the mortality of cervical cancer. Cervical cancer is a largely preventable malignancy with a long lead time. Vaccines for HPV have recently developed and are likely to help prevent infection with this frequently occurring sexually transmitted disease.

Treatment

Local ablative measures such as cryosurgery, laser ablation, or loop excision followed by regular screening surveillance.

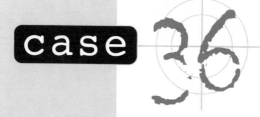

case 36

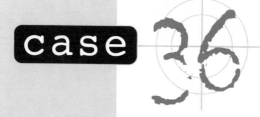

ID/CC	A 29-year-old **Vietnamese female** visits her family doctor because of protracted **nausea, vaginal bleeding, dyspnea, and hemoptysis.**
HPI	Her history reveals one previous normal gestation and one spontaneous abortion as well as a dilatation and curettage 4 months ago for a **hydatidiform mole.**
PE	Vaginal examination with speculum reveals **bluish-red vascular tumor** and **enlarged uterus**; adnexa and ovaries normal.
Labs	**Markedly elevated** serum and urinary **hCG levels.**
Imaging	CXR: **multiple metastatic nodules** ("CANNONBALL" SECONDARY LESIONS).
Micro Pathology	Exaggerated trophoblastic (cytotrophoblastic and syncytiotrophoblastic) tissue proliferation with endometrial penetration; cellular atypia and hematogenous/lymphatic spread.

GYNECOLOGY

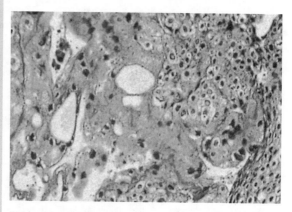

Figure 36-1. Multinucleated syncytiotrophoblasts with vacuolated cytoplasm adjacent to sheet of smaller mononuclear cytotrophoblasts.

71

case

Gestational Choriocarcinoma

Differential

Ectopic Pregnancy

Abortion

Hydatidiform Mole

Pulmonary Embolism

Metastatic Cancer

Discussion

Choriocarcinoma is a malignant gestational tumor that may develop during normal pregnancy, after evacuation of hydatidiform mole, or after previous spontaneous abortions. Patients have a uterus which is smaller than predicted gestational age with a dramatically elevated hCG. Choriocarcinoma can arise from gonadal neoplasms in both males and females and the prognosis is significantly worse if the tumor does not arise from a gestational product.

Treatment

Patients are treated with methotrexate (MTX) or Actinomycin D. Additional agents are employed with metastasis; follow-up with serial serum hCG levels.

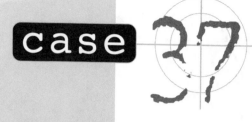

ID/CC A 33-year-old Hispanic **multigravida** in her 20th week of pregnancy comes to the gynecologist's office complaining of a **mass in her abdomen.**

HPI She is **pregnant for the fifth time.** She has had no prior abortions or C-sections.

PE VS: BP normal. PE: no edema; uterus correct height for gestational age (at level of umbilicus); **ill-defined, painless, nonmovable mass** 5 cm from midline on mesogastrium; skin not red or warm; no exudate; no fluctuation; **mass seems to disappear on contraction of rectus muscle.**

Labs Routine lab work on blood; urine and stool normal.

Imaging CT/MR, abdomen: circumscribed mass.

Gross Pathology Coarsely trabeculated tumor resembling scar tissue; appears to **arise from musculoaponeurotic wall.**

Micro Pathology Elongated, spindle-shaped cells; fibroblastic process; no evidence of atypical mitoses on biopsy.

GYNECOLOGY

case

Desmoid Tumor

Differential

Recurrent Germ Cell Tumor
Residual Mature Teratoma
Sarcomatoid Degeneration
Fibrosarcoma
Schwannoma

Discussion

A type of fibromatosis of the anterior abdominal wall in women, desmoid tumor is associated with previous trauma and multiple pregnancies. It occurs in increased frequency in Gardner's syndrome, a familial syndrome associated with mutations in the APC gene. It **frequently recurs after excision.**

Treatment

Wide surgical excision; radiotherapy for recurrent disease. Radiation therapy can be considered in recurrent cases or in patients who are poor surgical candidates.

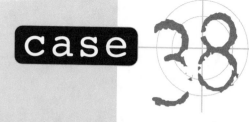

ID/CC A 16-year-old girl is seen with complaints of **colicky lower abdominal pain** together with nausea and vomiting associated with the **onset of menses**.

HPI She achieved menarche at 14, and her initial cycles were irregular but painless (due to anovulation). She does not complain of menstrual irregularity or excessive bleeding and has no urinary complaints or diarrhea.

PE Abdominal exam normal; gynecologic exam reveals blood-stained pad; pelvic exam not performed due to intact hymen; rectal exam normal.

Labs Routine lab parameters normal.

GYNECOLOGY

case

Primary Dysmennorrhea

Differential
Endometriosis
Inflammatory Bowel Disease
Irritable Bowel Syndrome
Pelvic Inflammatory Disease
Ovarian Cyst
Urinary Tract Infection

Discussion
Primary dysmenorrhea is defined as **painful periods** for which no organic or psychological cause can be found. Diagnosis is made on the basis of clinical findings. The pain is colicky and usually begins shortly after or at the onset of menses; it is thought to be due to an increase in the production of prostaglandins, leading to uterine vasoconstriction and painful contractions. Occurring **only during ovulatory cycles**, primary dysmenorrhea is most commonly found in women under the age of 20.

Treatment
Symptomatic relief with **prostaglandin synthetase inhibitors** such as mefenamic acid or naproxen sodium; intractable symptoms may require **suppression of ovulation** using combined estrogen/ progesterone or progestogens.

■ TABLE 38-1 CAUSES OF SECONDARY AMENORRHEA

Pregnancy	Menopause
Hypothyroidism	Hypothalamic amenorrhea
Anovulation	Asherman's syndrome
Premature ovarian failure	Pituitary Prolactin-secreting adenoma
Radiation/chemotherapy	Anorexia
Post oral contraceptive/	Exercise
Depo-Provera ammenorhea	

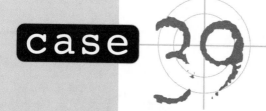

case 39

ID/CC	A 60-year-old **obese, nulliparous** white **female** presents with intermittent **postmenopausal vaginal bleeding** of 3 months' duration.
HPI	She has a history of **diabetes, hypertension,** and **infertility with polycystic ovaries;** menopause began at 56 years of age.
PE	**Uterus is not enlarged** on bimanual palpation.
Labs	CBC: mild anemia. Stool and urine tests within normal limits; endometrial biopsy diagnostic.
Imaging	US: pelvis: **thickening** of **endometrial stripe.**
Micro Pathology	Pap smear shows a cluster of medium sized malignant cells with eccentric nuclei and abnormally distributed chromatid.

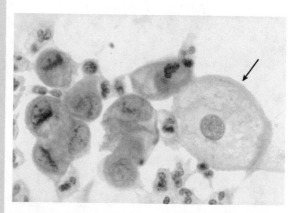

Figure 39-1. Medium sized malignant cells with eccentric nuclei and abnormally distributed chromatid. The arrow depicts a benign squamous cell.

case

Endometrial Carcinoma

Differential

Endometrial Hyperplasia

Endometrial Polyp

Endometrial Sarcoma

Cervical Carcinoma

Leiomyoma

Endometrial Atrophy

Discussion

Endometrial carcinoma is the most common gynecologic malignancy. It is associated with hyperestrogenic states, and depth of myometrial invasion is an important prognostic factor. Postmenopausal bleeding should be considered to be secondary to endometrial cancer until proven otherwise.

Risk factors for the development of endometrial cancer include: prolonged **estrogen stimulation** (as in hormone replacement), **obesity** (with increased peripheral conversion of androgens to estrogens), **diabetes,** and hypertension.

Treatment

Radiation therapy; hysterectomy; chemotherapy.

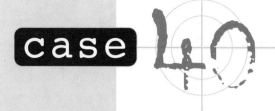
case 40

ID/CC A 27-year-old white female is admitted to the **infertility clinic** for evaluation of her **inability to conceive**; she also complains of **pain during intercourse** (DYSPAREUNIA) and **pain during menses** (DYSMENORRHEA).

HPI She is **nulligravida**. She admits to having **rectal pain during menstruation**; she also complains of having an **abundant menstrual period** (MENORRHAGIA OR HYPERMENORRHEA).

PE **Bluish spots in posterior fornix** on vaginal speculum exam; on bimanual exam, **fixed, tender bilateral ovarian masses palpable** during menstruation; **induration in pouch of Douglas** with **multiple small nodules** palpable through posterior fornix.

Labs CBC: mild anemia; normal WBC count. ESR normal.

Imaging Laparoscopy, pelvis: ovaries adhere to broad ligament and show retraction and scarring in addition to **"powder burn lesions,"** with dense peritubal and periovarian **adhesions** and **thickening of uterosacral ligaments**; biopsy of suspected lesions is taken. US: pelvis: nonspecific cystic enlargement of ovaries.

Gross Pathology Brownish nodules on uterosacral ligaments, ovaries, and pouch of Douglas.

Micro Pathology Laparoscopic biopsy of affected areas shows nodules consisting of endometrial glands, stroma, and hemosiderin pigment.

case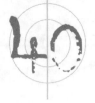

Endometriosis

Differential | Acute Appendicitis
Diverticular Disease
Ovarian Cyst
Pelvic Inflammatory Disease
Ectopic Pregnancy
Urinary Tract Infection

Discussion | Endometriosis refers to endometrial tissue that is present outside the uterus and produces symptoms that vary with location. It is the most common cause of chronic pelvic pain in women. Endometrial implants (endometriomas or **"chocolate cysts"**) most frequently involve both **ovaries**.

Treatment | Pain control with NSAIDs or opioids; alter hormonal environment with oral contraceptives, GnRH agonists, or danazol; if medical therapy fails, laparoscopic removal/coagulation of lesions or hysterectomy.

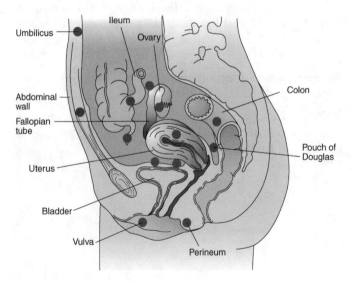

Figure 40-1. Common sites of endometriosis.

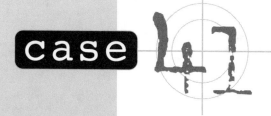
ID/CC A 42-year-old Filipina in her **20th week of pregnancy** presents with **vaginal bleeding but no pain.**

HPI She has been feeling inordinately **nauseated** and has suffered from ringing in her ears.

PE VS: moderate hypertension (BP 150/95). **Uterus large for gestational age** (three finger breadths above umbilicus); lower extremity 2+ **nonpitting edema.**

Labs **Markedly increased β-hCG.** UA: **proteinuria** but no casts seen on microscopic exam. Elevated blood uric acid level.

Imaging US: pelvis: complex **"snowstorm" appearance** and **no fetal parts** in uterine cavity.

Gross Pathology Characteristic appearance of **clusters of grapes.**

Micro Pathology Chorionic villi markedly enlarged and hydropic with surrounding cyto- and syncytiotrophoblastic tissue proliferation and lack of adequate vascular supply.

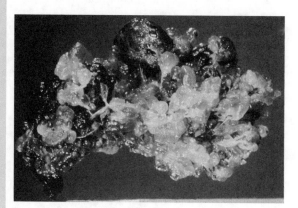

Figure 41-1. "Cluster of grapes".

case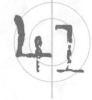

Hydatidiform Mole

Differential | Normal Pregnancy
Choriocarcinoma
Hyperemesis Gravidarum
Hypertension
Hypothyroidism

Discussion | A gestational neoplasm that may present as painless vaginal bleeding, **preeclampsia** in the first trimester, or **hyperemesis** gravidarum, hydatidiform mole may develop into **malignant choriocarcinoma** (20%). Hydatidiform mole is more common among females at extremes of reproductive age. Karyotypic analysis of a complete mole, which results from the fertilization of an ovum without a nucleus by a sperm, which subsequently duplicates its chromosome, is diploid XX. The karyotype of a partial mole, resulting from the fertilization of a normal ovum by 2 sperm, is triploid XXY or XXX. **Fetal parts are found in partial moles** although not in complete moles.

Treatment | Dilatation and suction curettage, periodic determination of hCG levels to identify development of invasive mole or choriocarcinoma.

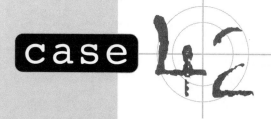

case 42

ID/CC	A **53-year-old female** complains of **increasing fatigue, insomnia, and depression.**
HPI	For the past 6 months she has had episodes in which her **face and neck have become hot and red** (HOT FLASHES). She has been **amenorrheic for the past 7 months;** prior to this, her menstrual history was normal.
PE	**Thinning of the skin; hirsutism; atrophic vaginal mucosa** with decreased secretions.
Labs	**Increased 24-hour urinary gonadotropins** (LH and FSH).
Imaging	DEXA: reveals osteoporosis. XR: plain: **osteoporosis** of thoracolumbar spine.

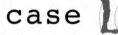

case 42

Menopause

Differential

Hypothyroidism
Polycystic Ovary Disease
Pituitary Adenoma
Pregnancy
Asherman Syndrome

Discussion

The estrogen deficiency state produced by menopause has short-range (hot flashes), medium-range (vaginal atrophy), and long-range (osteoporosis) consequences that can be relieved or prevented by estrogen replacement. Common side effects in patients taking hormone replacement therapy include irregular bleeding, weight gain, fluid retention, and endometrial hyperplasia. Nevertheless, postmenopausal bleeding should be worked up with an endometrial biopsy to rule out endometrial cancer.

Treatment

Treat osteoporosis with **bisphosphonates, calcitonin,** or selective estrogen receptor modulators; **estrogens** indicated for management of **vasomotor symptoms.**

■ TABLE 42-1 MANIFESTATIONS OF ESTROGEN DEFICIENCIES IN MENOPAUSAL WOMEN

Symptoms of Menopause	
Dyspareunia	Urinary urgency
Hot flushes	Night sweats
Pruritus due to vulvar, introital, and vaginal atrophy	Compression fractures Tooth loss
Skin atrophy	Vaginal dryness

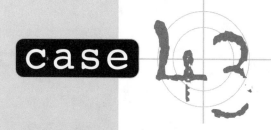

case 43

ID/CC	A **56-year-old white nulliparous woman** is referred for evaluation of a **pelvic mass** found on a routine physical.
HPI	She reports **increased frequency of micturition** and **irregular periods** until they ceased 3 years ago. **She has a history of breast cancer in the distant past.**
PE	**Large cystic mass** the size of a grapefruit in right pelvis that can be felt above the pubis symphysis.
Labs	**CA-125 levels elevated;** LFTs normal.
Imaging	CT/US: pelvis: **cystic pelvic mass arising out of right ovary.**
Gross Pathology	Partly solid and partly cystic mass.
Micro Pathology	Papillary structures of ciliated columnar cells; **psammoma bodies.**

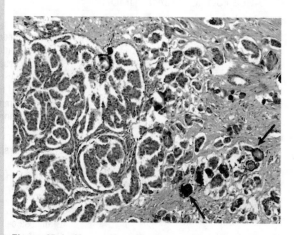

Figure 43-1. Abnormal ovarian tissue with several psammoma bodies (arrows).

85

case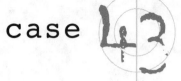

Serous Cystadenocarcinoma of the Ovaries

Differential	Ascites
	Irritable Bowel Syndrome
	Ovarian Cyst
	Pancreatic Cancer
	Rectal Cancer
Discussion	Ovarian cancer is the second most common gynecologic cancer; the **serous type** is **most common** and is **often bilateral.** It is often advanced at the time of diagnosis (omental masses, liver masses, ascites).
Treatment	Surgical staging and resection; chemotherapy; radiation therapy.

■ TABLE 43-1 OVARIAN TUMORS

Tumor Origin	Tumor Type
Surface epithelial tumors	Serous cystadenoma
	Serous cystadenocarcinoma
	Mucinous cystadenoma
	Mucinous cystadenocarcinoma
	Endometroid tumor
	Clear cell tumor
	Brenner tumor
Germ cell	Dysgerminoma
	Endodermal sinus (yolk sac) tumor
	Teratomas
	Ovarian choriocarcinoma
Ovarian sex cord-stromal origin	Fibroma
	Thecoma
	Granulosa cell tumor
	Sertoli-Leydig cell tumor
Metastasis to the ovary	

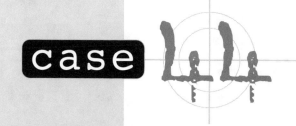

ID/CC	A 20-year-old Asian **female** visits her family doctor because of **chronic, intermittent left lower quadrant pain.**
HPI	The pain is not accompanied by dyspareunia, menstrual irregularity, vaginal discharge, abdominal distention, nausea, vomiting, or diarrhea. It is not correlated with her menstrual periods.
PE	**Left adnexal mass** on bimanual exam; uterosacral ligaments normal; pouch of Douglas normal; McBurney's point nontender; no evidence of ascites.
Labs	Routine lab work on blood, urine, and stool normal; CA-125 levels not elevated.
Imaging	US: pelvis: **large (5-cm) mass in left ovary.**
Micro Pathology	Vaginal smears for cytohormonal evaluation reveal excessive estrogenic stimulation and lack of progestational effect.
Gross Pathology	Large, sometimes multiple cystic structures on the ovary

GYNECOLOGY

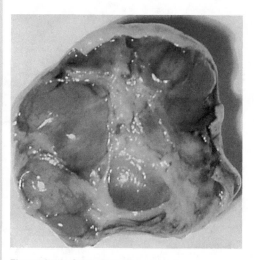

Figure 44-1. Gross Pathology sample.

87

case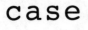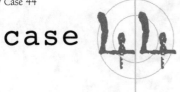

Ovarian Cyst—Follicular

Differential
Abdominal Abscess
Ectopic Pregnancy
Diverticulosis
Hydrosalpinx
Tubo-ovarian Abscess

Discussion
Most ovarian cysts are benign. Follicular ovarian cyst is the most common cause of ovarian enlargement.

Treatment
Follow-up by ultrasound (sizable percentage disappear spontaneously); laparoscopic removal if persistent.

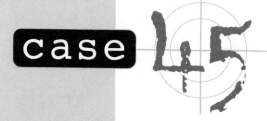

ID/CC A **25-year-old woman** complains of **loss of weight** and intense right lower abdominal pain and nausea that began when she went jogging yesterday afternoon.

HPI Intermittent episodes of similar pain have occurred over the past several days. She has regular menstrual cycles with average flow and no dysmenorrhea and had her last period 3 weeks ago.

PE VS: mild hypotension; normal HR (HR 90). PE: **right lower quadrant tenderness**; pelvic exam reveals tender, mobile 6-cm **right adnexal mass**.

Labs CBC: normal; pregnancy test negative.

Imaging XR: KUB: irregular **calcified** mass in region of right ovary. US: pelvis: **cystic tumor** about 8 cm in diameter replacing the right ovary.

Gross Pathology Cystic mass replacing the right ovary; thin, **fibrous wall with solid nodule at one aspect containing sebaceous material and matted hair;** tooth structures also seen.

GYNECOLOGY

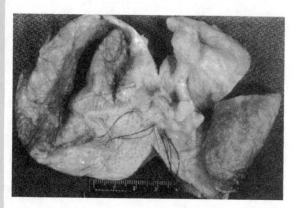

Figure 45-1. Surgical gross pathology specimen

case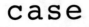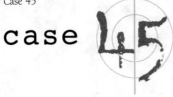

Ovarian Teratoma

Differential
Ovarian Cyst
Endometriosis
Germ Cell Tumor of the Ovary
Tubo-ovarian Abscess
Uterine Fibroid
Ectopic Pregnancy
Kidney

Discussion
Primary benign teratomas or dermoid cysts originate from germ cells; tumors are cystic and contain elements of all three germ cell layers. Complications of teratomas include torsion, infection, rupture leading to chemical peritonitis, infertility, secretion of thyroid hormone leading to hyperthyroidism (STRUMA OVARII), and carcinoid syndrome due to serotonin secretion; rarely, squamous cell carcinoma may develop in a dermoid cyst. Mature tissue elements **representing all three germ cell layers** are present, including skin with adnexal structures, bone, cartilage, teeth, thyroid, bronchi, intestine, and neural tissue.

Treatment
Surgical resection curative.

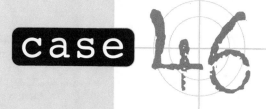

case 46

ID/CC   A **23-year-old** married **woman** is seen with complaints of **inability to conceive** after a year of unprotected intercourse (INFERTILITY).

HPI   Her last menstrual period was 3 months ago, and since menarche she **has only had 4 to 5 periods each year** (OLIGOMENORRHEA); a pregnancy test at home was negative. She also complains of **excessive facial hair**. Her **father was diabetic**.

PE   Patient **obese**; excessive **facial hair and male-pattern hair distribution on rest of body** (HIRSUTISM) but no virilization; pelvic exam normal; secondary sexual characteristics well developed.

Labs   **Elevated LH; decreased FSH** and loss of normal periodicity (LH: FSH, 3:1 ratio); **serum testosterone and androstenedione elevated; serum estradiol** (total and free) within normal limits in early and mid-follicular phases; **pattern of secretion abnormal with no preovulatory or midluteal increase**; TSH and prolactin levels normal.

Gross Pathology   Ovaries enlarged with **pearly-white capsule** and multiple cysts averaging 1 cm in diameter within stroma.

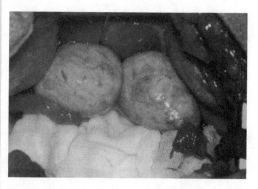

Figure 46-1. Note the large size of the ovaries, relative to the uterus, with a smooth ovarian capsule.

case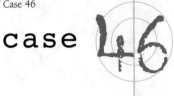

Polycystic Ovarian Syndrome

Differential
Androgen Producing Ovarian Tumors
Acromegaly
Cushing Syndrome
Hyperprolactinemia
Hypothyroidism

Discussion
Polycystic ovarian syndrome (**Stein–Leventhal syndrome**) is a clinical syndrome of **obesity, hirsutism, and secondary amenorrhea or oligomenorrhea with infertility due to anovulation,** accompanied by multiple-follicle cysts within both ovaries. PCOS patients are at increased risk for breast and endometrial carcinomas (due to unopposed LH stimulation).

Treatment
Reduce weight through diet and exercise; ovulation induction with clomiphene; laparoscopic ovarian diathermy or laser drilling in drug-resistant cases; low-dose combined contraceptive pill if contraception is desired.

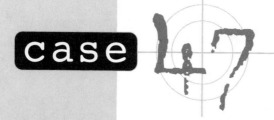

case 47

ID/CC A 17-year-old white **female** visits her family physician because she **has never had a menstrual period** (PRIMARY AMENORRHEA) and **lacks breast development.**

HPI She has a history of **low birth weight** and lymphedema of the hands and feet.

PE **Short stature;** low-set ears; **webbed neck;** cubitus valgus; low hairline; **shield-like chest with widely spaced nipples; harsh systolic murmur heard on back** (due to coarctation of aorta); hypoplastic nails; short fourth metacarpals; high-arched palate; **absence of pubic and axillary hair;** small clitoris and uterus; ovaries not palpable.

Labs High serum and urine FSH and LH; **no Barr bodies** on buccal smear. Karyotype: **45,XO.**

Imaging US: pelvis: infantile streak ovaries. Echo: bicuspid aortic valve.

Gross Pathology Fibrotic and atrophic ovaries.

Micro Pathology Absence of follicles in ovaries; normal ovarian stroma replaced by **fibrous streaks.**

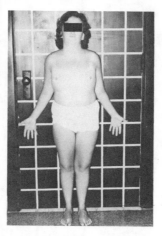

Figure 47-1. Patient on presentation.

case

Primary Amenorrhea—Turner Syndrome

Differential

Noonan Syndrome

Autoimmune Thyroiditis

Gonadal Dysgenesis

Lymphedema

Discussion

The most common karyotype is 45,XO; less common is mosaicism. Turner syndrome is associated with frequent skeletal, renal (horseshoe kidney), and cardiovascular anomalies (coarctation of the aorta) as well as with hypothyroidism.

Treatment

Growth hormone and androgens for increase in stature; subsequent estrogen therapy to protect against osteoporosis.

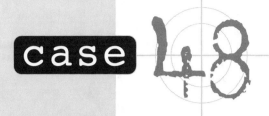

case 48

ID/CC	A 39-year-old **black female** presents with a several-month-long history of **profuse menstruation** (HYPERMENORRHEA) **and frequent menstrual periods** (POLYMENORRHEA).
HPI	Further questioning also reveals **painful periods** (DYSMENORRHEA) and increasing **urinary frequency.** She has a history of **infertility** and **recurrent spontaneous abortions.**
PE	**Enlarged, irregular uterus** on bimanual palpation with several masses on posterior wall.
Labs	CBC/PBS: hypochromic, microcytic anemia.
Imaging	US: pelvis: **multiple heterogeneous masses** distorting uterus.
Gross Pathology	Occur in myometrium (95% are intramural) and are round, firm, and well circumscribed.
Micro Pathology	Interlacing bundles of uniform, differentiated, elongated smooth muscle cells with few mitoses and no anaplasia; malignant transformation rare.

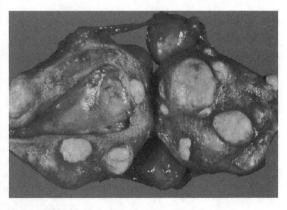

Figure 48-1. Multiple firm circumscribed, homogenous, yellowish nodules in the myometrium and protruding into endometrial cavity.

95

case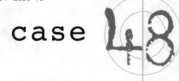

Uterine Fibroids

Differential

Endometrioma
Dermoid
Adenomyosis
Malignant Ovarian Tumors
Pregnancy

Discussion

The **most common tumor of the uterus** and the **most common tumor in women,** uterine fibroids are **estrogen-dependent** and commonly occur after 30 years of age; they tend to regress after menopause unless the patient is on hormone replacement therapy.

Treatment

Myomectomy; hysterectomy; gonadotropin-releasing hormone analogs; embolization by interventional radiology.

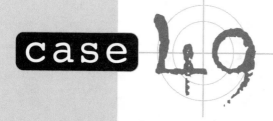
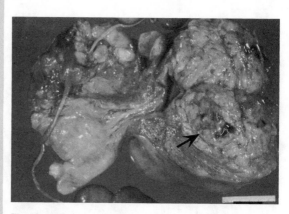

ID/CC	A 60-year-old woman visits her gynecologist because of a **foul-smelling, blood-tinged, purulent vaginal discharge.**
HPI	She has never been married and **has never been pregnant.** She is hypertensive and takes oral hypoglycemic agents for diabetes mellitus.
PE	VS: BP normal at present. PE: overweight; **fleshy, bulky, fungating tumor** protruding from cervical os on vaginal speculum exam.
Imaging	CT/MR: large, complex mass arising from uterus.
Gross Pathology	Large, fleshy tumor of myometrium with areas of necrosis and hemorrhage.
Micro Pathology	Background of spindle-shaped cells with **more than 10 mitoses per high-power field** on biopsy; many mitoses have abnormal mitotic spindle.

GYNECOLOGY

Figure 49-1. Large fleshy tan mass in the mymetrium with areas of hemorrhage softening and focal necrosis.

97

case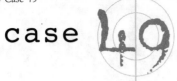

Uterine Leiomyosarcoma

Differential

Uterine Fibroid
Dermoid
Adenomyosis
Malignant Ovarian Tumors

Discussion

A highly aggressive malignant tumor of myometrium, leiomyosarcoma of the uterus may arise in a leiomyoma or de novo. It spreads by contiguity, hematogenously, and through lymphatics.

Treatment

Adriamycin, progestins, combination chemotherapy. Surgical therapy (total abdominal hysterectomy with bilateral salpingo-oophorectomy, or TAH-BSO) with adjuvant chemotherapy or radiation therapy.

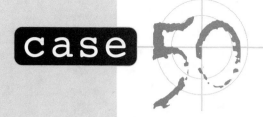

case 50

ID/CC	A **65-year-old woman** is referred for intractable vulvar growth and **pruritus**.
HPI	She has also felt an obstruction in the flow of her urine. She was a **prostitute** and was treated often for STDs. She is a **chronic smoker**.
PE	Gynecologic exam reveals excoriation marks over vulva; exophytic growth arising from left labia majora; left inguinal lymphadenopathy.
Labs	Cystoscopy reveals lower urethral stenosis (due to involvement by vulvar growth).
Gross Pathology	Gross examination reveals firm, exophytic growth.

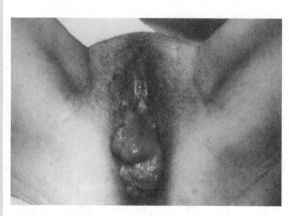

Figure 50-1. Exophytic vulvar neoplasm.

case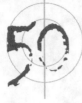

Vulvar Carcinoma

Differential

Vulvar Atrophy
Vulvovaginitis
Lichen Sclerosis
Lichen Planus
Squamous Hyperplasia
Paget's Disease of the Vulva
Eczema

Discussion

Vulvar cancer is a disease of **older women** with a mean age of 65 years. It is associated with **smoking**, and its recent increase in incidence among younger women is associated with **papillomavirus.** Carcinoma in situ (vulvar intraepithelial neoplasia, or VIN) and squamous dysplasia are considered precursor lesions. **Cloquet's node** indicates distant metastases.

Treatment

Confirm diagnosis with biopsy; preoperative radiotherapy to shrink tumor mass; radical vulvectomy with lymph node dissection.

case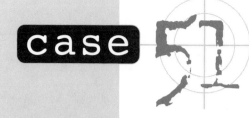

ID/CC A 75-year-old white **woman** visits her gynecologist for a routine checkup and is found to have **white spots** on her **genitalia**.

HPI She complains of slight outer vaginal **itching** but denies any postmenopausal bleeding, vaginal discharge, or drug intake.

PE **Hypochromic macules** on labia majora extending to perineum and inner thighs in patchy distribution with **scale formation** (DESQUAMATION); **skin thickened and rough** (HYPERKERATOTIC); no regional lymphadenopathy; atrophic vaginitis on vaginal speculum exam.

Micro Pathology Biopsy reveals hyperkeratosis and fibrosis with thinning of squamous epithelium; lymphocytic inflammatory infiltration, most prevalent surrounding blood vessels; no chronic inflammatory response; no signs of malignant transformation.

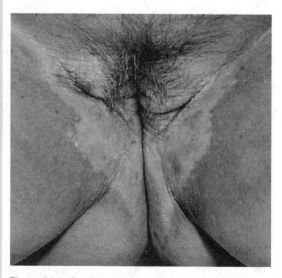

Figure 51-1. Sharply demarcated white plaque-like lesions on the vulva.

101

case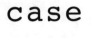

Vulvar Leukoplakia

Differential	Lichen Planus
	Lichen Sclerosis
	Vitiligo
	Squamous Hyperplasia
	Vulvar Carcinoma
Discussion	**Vulvar leukoplakia** is a clinical diagnosis that can be attributed to a variety of disorders that all produce white patches. Causes may be benign disorders such as vitiligo, as well as inflammatory conditions, pre-malignant conditions (e.g., dystrophies), or squamous cell carcinoma. **Always perform a biopsy.**
Treatment	**Biopsy;** subsequent treatment dependent on diagnosis. Treat with topical steroids unless malignancy is found.

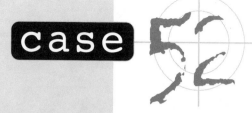

case 52

ID/CC	A **73-year-old** woman is brought to a gynecologist by her daughter, who became aware of a **genital ulcer** while helping her mother shower.
HPI	Her history reveals **weight loss** and **dyspnea** together with hypertension and arthritis.
PE	Hard, nodular, 5-mm **pigmented and ulcerated** lesion on upper right **labia minora;** no inguinal lymphadenopathy; scattered crepitant rales on chest auscultation.
Labs	CBC/PBS: slight anemia.
Imaging	CXR: **multiple metastatic nodules.**
Micro Pathology	Biopsy reveals cells with lymphocytic reaction infiltrating into underlying dermis; cells stain **positive for S100 antigen** and are **negative for mucin.**

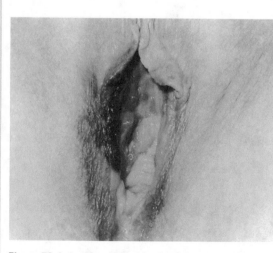

Figure 52-1. Lesion of the vulva involving the right labia minora.

OBSTETRICS

case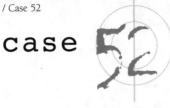

Vulvar Malignant Melanoma

Differential

Vulvar Atrophy

Lichen Sclerosis

Vitiligo

Squamous Hyperplasia

Vulvar Carcinoma

Paget Disease of the Vulva

Discussion

Vulvar malignant melanoma is the second most common vulvar malignancy (the first is squamous cell carcinoma); metastasis and prognosis depend on the extent of vertical growth.

Treatment

Surgery with regional lymph node dissection and adjuvant chemotherapy.

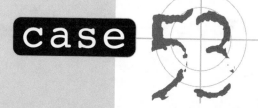

case 53

ID/CC	A 25-year-old **woman** presents with **amenorrhea** of 6 weeks' duration and **pelvic pain** over the past day.
HPI	She has a history of **vaginal spotting off and on** for the past 2 weeks and has been using an **IUD** for the past 3 years. She has no history of vaginal discharge and no urinary symptoms, and her previous menstrual history is normal. She has had multiple bouts of **pelvic inflammatory disease**.
PE	VS: BP normal. PE: pallor; abdominal distention and decreased bowel sounds; **cervical motion tenderness**; uterus soft and slightly enlarged on pelvic exam; **soft, tender, boggy mass in right adnexa and pouch of Douglas.**
Labs	CBC: anemia. **hCG levels lower than expected** for this period of gestation; culdocentesis reveals presence of blood in cul-de-sac.
Imaging	US: pelvis: **no products of conception in uterine cavity;** doughnut-shaped mass in right adnexa; echogenic free fluid in cul-de-sac.
Gross Pathology	Pending
Micro Pathology	Uterine curettage reveals presence of Arias–Stella reaction in the **absence of villi.**

OBSTETRICS

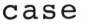 case

Ectopic Pregnancy

Differential	Spontaneous Abortion
	Appendicitis
	Pelvic Inflammatory Disease
	Endometriosis
Discussion	Other risk factors for ectopic pregnancy include **previous tubal surgery**, tubal ligation, **endometriosis, previous ectopic pregnancy,** and ovulation induction.
Treatment	Laparoscopic linear salpingostomy and segmental resection; methotrexate for selected cases without signs of active bleeding or hemoperitoneum.

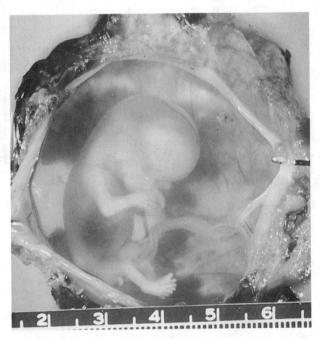

Figure 53-1. An enlarged fallopian tube has been opened to expose a minute fetus.

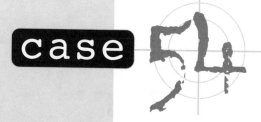

ID/CC	A 38-year-old **grand multipara** develops a marked drop in her blood pressure following **uncontrolled bleeding immediately after delivery.**
HPI	She delivered **twins** at 35 weeks' gestation with **polyhydramnios.**
PE	VS: **hypotension; tachycardia.** PE: anxious; pallor; low central venous pressure; **uterus soft and flabby** with indistinct outline.
Labs	CBC: anemia; mildly decreased hematocrit. Coagulation profile normal.
Gross Pathology	Uterus **grossly overdistended and flabby.**

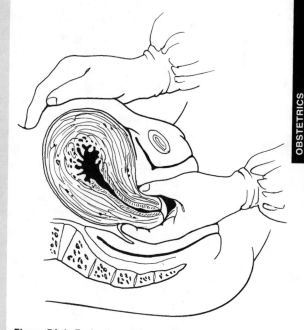

Figure 54-1. Evaluation of the postpartum uterus.

case

Postpartum Hemorrhage

Differential

Uterine Rupture
Uterine Inversion
Retained Placenta
Uterine Atony
Vaginal Laceration
Coagulopathy

Treatment

Fluid resuscitation; blood transfusion; uterine massage; maintain contraction with an oxytocin infusion; ergotamine for vasoconstriction; if found, **remove retained placenta;** check for cervical, vaginal, or uterine lacerations and uterine rupture; hypogastric artery ligation and/or hysterectomy if other measures fail.

Discussion

Primary postpartum hemorrhage (PPH) is defined as loss of 500 mL or more of blood within 24 hours of a vaginal delivery (1000 mL after a C-section) or any amount of bleeding that is sufficient to produce a hemodynamic compromise; primary causes include uterine atony, retained placenta, and soft tissue injury. Factors associated with an increased risk of uterine atony and retained placenta include **high multiparity, a maternal age greater than 35 years, delivery after an antepartum hemorrhage, multiple pregnancies, polyhydramnios, a past history of PPH, and coagulation disorders.** Sheehan's syndrome—a clinical syndrome of hypopituitarism secondary to ischemic pituitary necrosis—is a peculiar complication of massive postpartum hemorrhage.

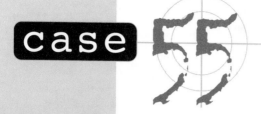

case 55

ID/CC	A 28-year-old **woman** presents with **swelling of her entire left leg** of 1 day's duration.
HPI	She delivered a normal full-term male baby 2 days ago.
PE	Low grade fever. Left leg **erythematous, warm, swollen** (greater than 2 cm in diameter than the contralateral leg), and **tender.** Pain and tenderness in the calf of the affected extremity, especially on dorsiflexion of the foot (Homan sign).
Labs	Routine tests normal; normal clotting profile.
Imaging	US: Doppler: clot in left femoral vein. Venography: confirmatory "gold standard" but usually not required.

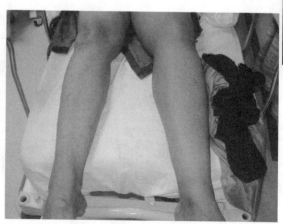

Figure 55-1. Lower extremity edema and erythema.

case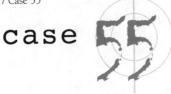

Postpartum Thrombophlebitis

Differential

Ruptured Baker's Cyst
Pulmonary Embolism
Lymphedema
Hematoma
Arterial Insufficiency
Varicose Veins

Discussion

Phlegmasia alba dolens (painful white leg) is due to iliofemoral vein thrombosis occurring in late pregnancy and **postpartum;** it is related to **compression by a gravid uterus** and **hypercoagulability** of pregnancy. Additional risk factors in this population include genetic mutations such as factor V Leiden, smoking, and use of oral contraceptives containing high doses of estrogen.

Treatment

IV heparin and monitoring of clotting time and PTT; elevation of limb; analgesics and soaks. Coagulation with low molecular weight heparin or Warfarin. Although contraindicated in pregnancy, Warfarin can be given to nursing mothers.

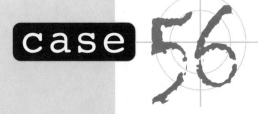

case 56

ID/CC	A 30-year-old **woman** presents with fatigue, **significant weight loss**, and **amenorrhea** of 2 years' duration.
HPI	She had a baby 2 years ago and suffered **significant postpartum bleeding.** She bottle-fed her baby because she was **unable to lactate** after delivery.
PE	VS: **hypotension** (BP 85/60). PE: skin tenting; fine wrinkling around eyes and mouth; loss of axillary and pubic hair.
Labs	**Decreased levels of trophic hormones (FSH, LH, ACTH, TSH, GH, prolactin);** decreased levels of target gland hormones (T_3, T_4, cortisol, estrogens).
Imaging	MR: pituitary (usually before and after injection of gadolinium DTPA): abnormal signal in pituitary gland.
Gross Pathology	Soft, pale, and hemorrhagic pituitary gland in early stages; shrunken, fibrous, and firm in later stages.

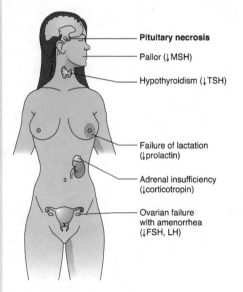

Figure 56-1. Patient on presentation.

OBSTETRICS

111

case

Sheehan's Syndrome

Differential
Empty Sella Syndrome
Pituitary Adenoma
Lyphocytic Hypophysitis

Discussion
Sheehan's syndrome is most commonly caused by **postpartum infarction of the pituitary.** During pregnancy, the anterior pituitary grows to nearly twice its normal size. During delivery, loss of blood or hypovolemia decreases flow to the pituitary, inducing vasospasm that leads to **ischemic necrosis** of the anterior pituitary. The posterior pituitary is supplied by arteries and is therefore much less susceptible to ischemia. Loss of trophic hormones leads to atrophy of target organs. Ischemic necrosis may also occur in males and in nonpregnant females (trauma, sickle cell anemia, disseminated intravascular coagulation, vascular accidents).

Treatment
Hormone replacement: cortisol; levothyroxine (T_4); estrogen-progesterone replacement.

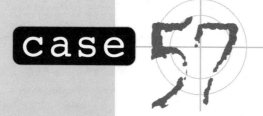

case 57

ID/CC A 30-year-old white **primigravida** at **36 weeks of gestation** visits her obstetrician for the first time in her pregnancy complaining of **swollen legs and headache.**

HPI Her medical history is unremarkable, and her pregnancy had apparently developed with no complications until the onset of her symptoms.

PE VS: **hypertension** (BP 170/110). PE: **excessive weight gain** (19 kg); funduscopic exam does not show changes of hypertensive retinopathy; 3+ **pitting pedal edema;** 1+ periorbital edema; fundal height appropriate; fetal parts palpable; fetal heart sounds normal.

Labs CBC/PBS: complete blood counts and coagulation profile normal. Serum uric acid concentrations raised; mildly elevated AST and ALT; 3+ **proteinuria.**

Imaging US: OB: single live fetus; lie longitudinal; presentation cephalic; normal biophysical profile; **placental infarctions** seen.

Micro Pathology Endothelial cell swelling with obliteration of glomerular capillary lumen on renal biopsy.

case

Toxemia of Pregnancy—Preeclampsia

Differential

Essential Hypertension

Graves' Disease

Thyroid Storm

Acute Renal Failure

Pheochromocytoma

Systemic Lupus Erythromatosis

Discussion

Preeclampsia occurs in 5% of all pregnancies; it is most common during the **last trimester of a first pregnancy.** It is characterized by the triad of **hypertension, proteinuria, and edema.** Progression to eclampsia may occur with visual disturbances, seizures, and coma. Other complications include DIC and HELLP syndrome (hemolysis, elevated LFTs, low platelets), which can cause severe liver dysfunction.

Treatment

Antihypertensive agents; delivery of fetus and placenta, usually by C-section.

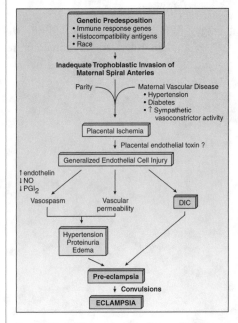

Figure 57-1. Pathogenesis of toxemia of pregnancy.

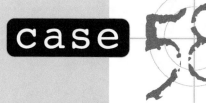

ID/CC	A 5-year-old **Asian** female develops **sudden,** acute **pain** and **loss of vision** in the right eye after watching a series of family slides in a **dark room.**
HPI	She had been complaining of seeing **"halos" around lights** at night.
PE	Injection (due to vasodilation) of ciliary and conjunctival blood vessels; **hazy cornea;** loss of peripheral vision; **markedly elevated intraocular pressure;** shallow anterior chamber with peripheral iridocorneal contact by slit-lamp exam; pupils mid-dilated and unresponsive to light and accommodation; hyperemic and edematous optic nerve bed on funduscopic exam.
Gross Pathology	Pathologically narrow anterior chamber; eye hyperopic and **rock-hard** in consistency; synechia formation; Schlemm's canal may be blocked.
Micro Pathology	Degeneration and fibrosis of trabeculae.

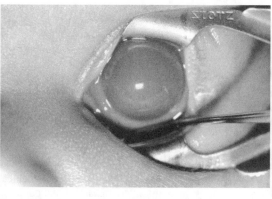

Figure 58-1. This cornea is diffusely opacified and enlarged.

case

Acute Closed Angle Glaucoma

Differential
Central Retinal Vein Occlusion

Choroidal Detachment

Conjunctivitis

Uveitis

Scleritis

Discussion
Acute angle-closure glaucoma is characterized by a sudden increase in intraocular pressure that may be **precipitated by mydriatics** and upon leaving **dark environments** for well-lit areas. The intraocular pressure represents a balance between the rate of formation of aqueous humor and the outflow of the chamber. In acute **closed angle glaucoma**, the peripheral iris touches the trabecular meshwork and blocks the flow of aqueous to the trabecular meshwork.

Treatment
Analgesics, IV acetazolamide; topical beta-blockers; steroids; pilocarpine; **laser iridotomy.**

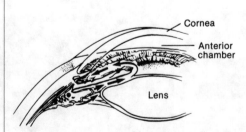

Figure 58-2. Normal anterior chamber angle. Aqueous passes from the posterior chamber through the pupil into the anterior chamber and out through the trabecular meshwork.

case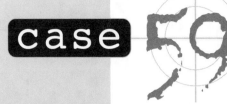

ID/CC   A 28-year-old **woman** presents with a sudden, severe attack of vertigo associated with nausea and vomiting.

HPI   Her symptoms begin and are aggravated when she looks toward the right. The attacks last less than 30 seconds. She has no history of hearing loss, ear discharge, tinnitus, trauma, pain, or restricted neck movement.

PE   Symptoms recur when her head is turned toward right; rotatory fatigable nystagmus with a linear component; no hearing loss or any other neurologic deficit. Patient experiences reproducible vertigo with **Dix-Hallpike Maneuver.**

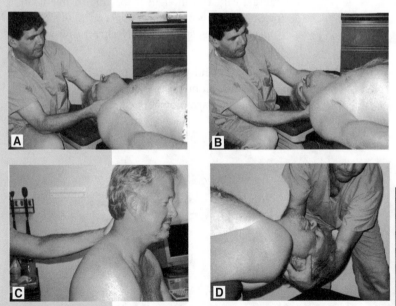

Figure 59-1. Patient supine, head over side of table (A). Extend patient's head at neck 25 to 30 degrees and rotate head to right or left for 30 seconds (B). Assist patient to rapidly assume a sitting position, maintain for 1 minute (C). Repeat the procedure with the head rotated to other side (D).

ENT/OPTHALMOLOGY

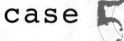

Benign Positional Vertigo

Differential

Labyrinthitis

Acute Otitis Media

Migraine Headache

Meniere's Disease

Drug Reaction

Acoustic Neuroma

Transient Ischemic Attack

Multiple Sclerosis

Ramsay-Hunt Syndrome

Discussion

Benign positional vertigo is sometimes seen after head injuries, ear operations, or infections of the middle ear; it is thought to be due to free-floating otoconial debris in the posterior semicircular canal. It typically abates spontaneously after a few weeks or months.

Treatment

Reassurance and positioning maneuvers designed to clear debris from the posterior canal. Meclizine or Diazepam for symptomatic relief.

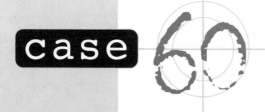

case 60

ID/CC   A 16-year-old male seen after a roadside accident presents with a **persistent bloody but thin nasal and ear discharge.**

HPI   The driver of the vehicle states that he saw the patient ejected from the vehicle and hit the back of his head on the pavement.

PE   Watery nasal discharge noted; **bilateral periorbital hematomas** ("raccoon eye") seen; perimastoid ecchymosis (Battle's sign); **anosmia** found on neurologic exam; on placing a drop of nasal discharge on clean white gauze, **spreading yellow halo noted in addition to central blood stain** (HALO SIGN; due to presence of CSF). Glasgow coma scale of 8.

Imaging Pending.

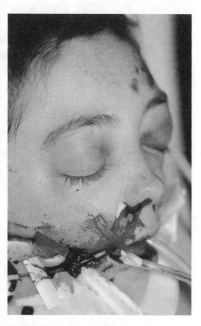

Figure 60-1. "Raccoon eyes".

case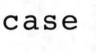

Basilar Skull Fracture

Differential

Cribriform Plate Fracture
Subdural Hematoma
Petrous Temporal Bone Fracture

Discussion

Fractures of the base of the skull involve the anterior or middle cranial fossa. Those affecting the anterior fossa, as in this case, may cause nasal bleeding, periorbital hematomas, subconjunctival hemorrhages, CSF rhinorrhea, and cranial nerve injuries (CN I–CN V); **middle cranial fossa structures involving the petrous temporal bone may cause bleeding from the ear, CSF otorrhea, bruising of the ear over the mastoid** (BATTLE SIGN), **and cranial nerve injuries** (CN VII–CN VIII).

Treatment

Antibiotics; head end elevated by 30 degrees; patient **advised not to blow his nose;** neurosurgical consult for possible repair of meninges. Seizure precautions.

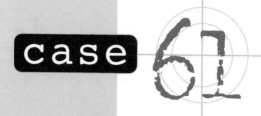

case 61

ID/CC	A **50-year-old male** complains of **hearing loss and a whistling sound in his left ear** (TINNITUS).
HPI	He claims to have pronounced **difficulty understanding speech** (out of proportion to hearing loss). He has also experienced occasional **vertigo**.
PE	Left-sided **sensorineural deafness; Weber test lateralized toward right ear;** left-sided corneal reflex lost (CN V dysfunction).
Labs	Pure-tone audiometry reveals sensorineural hearing loss; **discrimination of speech markedly reduced;** loudness recruitment absent; tone decay seen.
Imaging	MR: left **cerebellopontine-angle** abnormality.
Gross Pathology	**Encapsulated tumor** arising out of periphery of CN VIII (vestibular division) at cerebellopontine angle.
Micro Pathology	**Spindle cells** with tightly interlaced pattern (ANTONI A) and **Verocay bodies**.

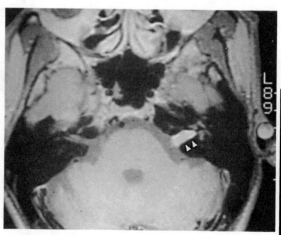

Figure 61-1. MR image demonstrating a tumor of the cerebellopontine angle.

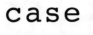
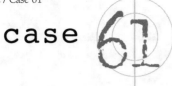

case 61

Acoustic Neuroma

Differential

Migraine Headache
Quinine Toxicity
Labyrinthitis
Vestibular Neuronitis
Meningioma
Meniere Disease

Discussion

These benign tumors arise from the distal neurilemmal portion of the 8th nerve, usually from the vestibular division, and are correctly called schwannomas; they account for **80% of cerebellopontine tumors.** Acoustic neuromas can be successfully removed, but cranial nerve palsies such as CN VII nerve and deafness are common. These tumors are associated with genetic disease neurofibromatosis I (unilateral acoustic neuromas) and II (bilateral acoustic neuromas).

Treatment

Micro-surgical resection; stereotactic radiosurgery.

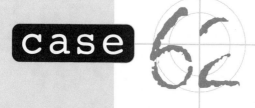

case 62

ID/CC   A 73-year-old female complains of sudden-onset **dizziness, nausea, vomiting (nonprojectile), and loss of balance.**

HPI   She also complains of hearing loss and tinnitus. She has **chronic suppurative otitis media** (CSOM) of the right ear, for which she has taken treatment irregularly.

PE   Patient lying on left ear and looking toward right ear; **conductive deafness;** Weber lateralized toward right ear in right ear; horizontal spontaneous nystagmus toward left; no neurologic deficits.

Imaging   MR: brain and right internal auditory canal: T1-weighted postcontrast images demonstrate enhancing cochlea, vestibule, and semicircular canals on right side. No evidence of brain abscess, neuroma, or cholesteatoma.

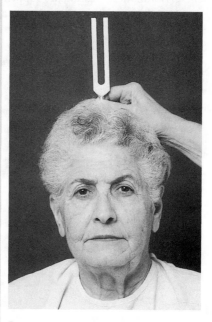

Figure 62-1. Weber test for lateralization of hearing loss.

case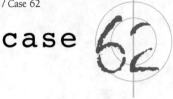

Labyrinthitis

Differential
Benign Positional Vertigo
Migraine Headache
Multiple Sclerosis
Vestibular Neuronitis
Transient Ischemic Attack
Meniere Disease

Discussion
Pyogenic inflammation of the labyrinth may result from acute otitis media, operations on the stapes, or preformed pathways such as fracture lines; in CSOM, cholesteatoma may cause erosion of the semicircular canals, exposing the labyrinth to infections. Meningitis is a serious complication of suppurative labyrinthitis.

Treatment
Antibiotics, vestibular suppressants, and surgical exploration with myringotomy and drainage.

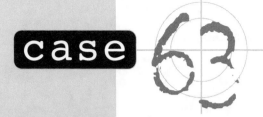

case 63

ID/CC A 45-year-old **obese** man presents with **excessive daytime sleepiness** that has progressively worsened over the past 3 years.

HPI His wife complains that his **snoring** can be heard in the adjacent room and that he intermittently appears to stop breathing during the night. These **"no-breathing" episodes** last 30 to 90 seconds, and then, with a loud snort, he begins to breathe again. The patient also reports fatigue, forgetfulness, anxiety, **morning headaches**, and diminished sexual interest.

PE VS: **mild hypertension** (140/90). PE: **short, thick neck; deviated nasal septum; pharyngeal crowding with enlarged, floppy uvula, high-arched palate, and soft palate resting on base of tongue.**

Labs Overnight pulse oximetry reveals **frequent episodes of arterial O_2 desaturation; polysomnography** (including EEG, ECG, eye movement, chin movement, air flow, chest and abdominal effort, SaO_2, snoring, and leg movement) **diagnostic.**

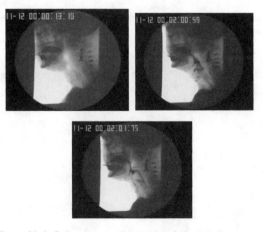

Figure 63-1. Polysomnographic tracing demonstrating obstructive apnea, mixed apnea, central apnea, and hypopnea.

case

Obstructive Sleep Apnea

Differential

Simple Snoring

Obesity Hypoventilation Syndrome (Pickwickian Syndrome)

Narcolepsy

Chronic Insufficient Sleep

Treatment

Weight loss; avoidance of alcohol and sedatives; **nasal CPAP** or BiPAP; pharmacotherapy with protryptiline; **surgical interventions** include uvulopalatopharyngoplasty (UPPP).

Discussion

Pathophysiologically, nasopharyngeal crowding creates a critical subatmospheric pressure during inspiration that overcomes the ability of the airway dilator and abductor muscles to maintain airway patency. This causes apnea, leading to hypoxemia that eventually arouses the patient from sleep. In patients with obstructive sleep apnea, there is an **increased incidence** of **coronary events, CVAs,** and **right heart failure.**

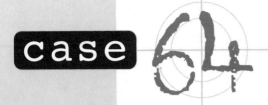

ID/CC A **44-year-old black male** is referred to the ophthalmologist for evaluation of **progressive** and **painless diminution of vision.**

HPI He has no known drug allergies and denies use of steroids.

PE VS: normal. PE: ophthalmology exam reveals normal visual acuity with markedly **reduced peripheral field of vision; elevated intraocular pressure** on tonometry; **increased cup-to-disk ratio with optic atrophy** on ophthalmoscopy; wide open angle noted on gonioscopy.

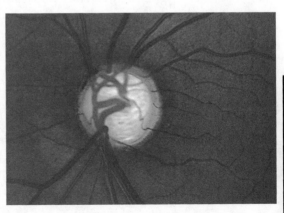

Figure 64-1. Clinical photograph of a glaucomatous optic disc with characteristic enlargement of the optic disc cup.

ENT/OPTHALMOLOGY

case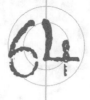

Open Angle Glaucoma

Differential | Chronic Closed Angle Glaucoma
Drug-induced Glaucoma
Ocular Ischemic Syndrome
Sturge-Weber Syndrome
Carotid Cavernous Fistula

Discussion | Open angle glaucoma is the **most frequent cause of vision loss in the African-American population.** **Risk factors** include **diabetes, nearsightedness,** and **long-term steroid** use. People with **first-degree relatives** with glaucoma are at increased risk. Unfortunately, the disease is usually far advanced when symptoms are first noted. Prevention is through early detection with eye exams once every 2 years or more frequently for those at increased risk.

Treatment | **Relief of intraocular hypertension** with topical beta-blockers (timolol), miotics (pilocarpine), or prostaglandin inhibitors with or without surgical procedures such as laser trabeculoplasty, trabeculotomy, goniotomy, and trabeculectomy.

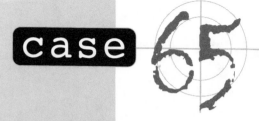

case 65

ID/CC	A **60-year-old male** complains of **progressively diminishing hearing acuity over the past few years.**
HPI	The patient's hearing loss is **bilateral** and is almost the **same for both ears;** he has no history of ear discharge, tinnitus, or trauma.
PE	Ability to distinguish between consonants markedly impaired; **air conduction exceeds bone conduction** (due to sensorineural hearing loss); audiometry reveals **bilateral hearing loss in higher-frequency range.**
Micro Pathology	Loss of hair cells, atrophy of the spinal ganglion, altered endolymph production, and thickening of the basilar membrane with some neural degeneration.

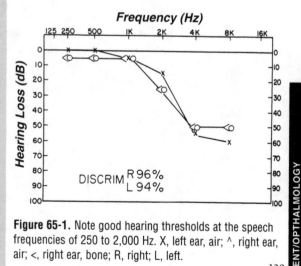

Figure 65-1. Note good hearing thresholds at the speech frequencies of 250 to 2,000 Hz. X, left ear, air; ^, right ear, air; <, right ear, bone; R, right; L, left.

case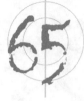

Presbycusis

Differential

Autoimmune Hearing Loss

Cholesteatoma

Chronic Otitis Media

Acoustic Neuroma

Otosclerosis

Treatment

Hearing aids with high-frequency gain, assistive listening devices, and cochlear implants.

Discussion

Presbycusis is a type of sensorineural hearing loss that results from the **aging process;** degenerative changes occur in the cells of the organ of Corti and nerve fibers. Deafness is bilateral and symmetrical, commonly **affecting the high tones.** Other types of presbycusis include strial, which starts in the fourth and sixth decades, is slowly progressive, and is characterized by good discrimination and by the presence of recruitment, a flat or descending audiogram, and patchy atrophy of the middle and apical turns of the stria. Cochlear deafness begins in middle age and is of the conductive variety, showing a downward slope on audiogram and absent pathologic findings. Both types of sensorineural loss can be avoided through use of protection in high-noise areas and monitoring of ototoxic drugs.

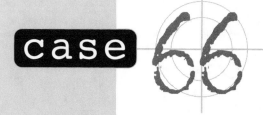

case 66

ID/CC A 45-year-old male is seen with complaints of **blurring of vision while reading and performing similar tasks involving near vision.**

HPI He complains that he has to hold the newspaper at an increasing distance in order to read it clearly. He has had no previous problems with his vision and has no history of diabetes or hypertension.

PE **Amplitude of accommodation reduced;** convex lens reduced near-point distance, allowing patient to read comfortably and to engage in tasks requiring near vision.

case

Presbyopia

Differential

Myopia

Hyperopia

Astigmatism

Diabetic Associated Lens Changes

Anisometropia

Discussion

Presbyopia is **natural loss of accommodation** due to **sclerosis of the lens substance,** which fails to adapt itself to a more spherical shape when the zonule is relaxed in the accommodation reflex. Presbyopia is seen in middle-aged patients (mean age 45 years).

Treatment

Convex lens glasses for work requiring near vision, contact lens, Conductive Keratoplasty (reshaping of the peripheral cornea with radio-frequency).

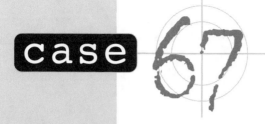
ID/CC	A 29-year-old woman visits a clinic with complaints of **visual blurring**.
HPI	She also complains of **headaches** that are worse in the morning. She has been taking **oral contraceptives** for some time.
PE	VS: BP normal. PE: patient is **obese;** funduscopy reveals presence of **papilledema;** no focal neurologic deficit noted; remainder of exam normal.
Labs	LP: elevated opening pressure; CSF normal.
Imaging	CT: ventricles normal, increased volume of subarachnoid spaces. MR venogram: rules out dural sinus thrombosis.

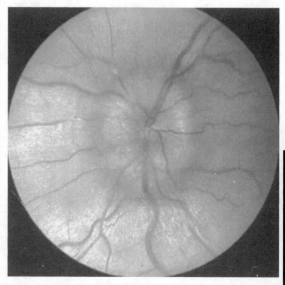

Figure 67-1. Patient with papilledema; there is swelling of the optic disk as a result of increased intracranial pressure. Note the loss of the central cup.

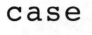

case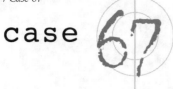

Pseudotumor Cerebri

Differential
Arteriovenous Malformation
Aseptic Meningitis
Hydrocephalus
Intracranial Hemorrhage
Intracranial Neoplasm
Migraine Headache
Meningioma

Discussion
Benign intracranial hypertension is primarily a disease of **obese females**; its etiology is unknown, although associations exist with the use of certain drugs (oral contraceptives, steroids, nalidixic acid, tetracycline) as well as with pregnancy, previous head injury, dural sinus thrombosis, and excessive vitamin A intake. Complications include progressive optic neuropathy leading to visual field constriction.

Treatment
Stop oral contraceptives; advise diuretics and obesity-reducing measures. If medical treatment becomes inadequate, surgical options such as shunt placement are used.

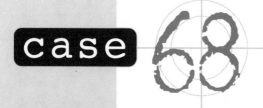
ID/CC   A **16-year-old male** is referred to an ophthalmologist for an evaluation of a **progressively constricting visual field.**

HPI   The boy complains that he sees as though he were looking **through a narrow tube.** Directed questioning reveals that he has a long-standing history of **night blindness** (due to loss of rods). His parents, although normal, had a **consanguineous marriage** and have a **family history of a visual disorder.**

PE   Funduscopy reveals "**bone spicule**" **pigmentation** in midperiphery of fundus, waxy appearance of optic disk, and marked narrowing and attenuation of vessels; **field of vision shows concentric contraction** that is especially marked if illumination is reduced.

Labs   **Electroretinogram and electro-oculogram demonstrate reduced activity.**

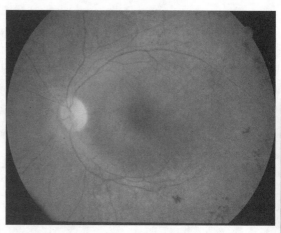

Figure 68-1. The optic nerve head is pale, the blood vessels are attenuated, and there is mild atrophy and bony black spicule formation in the periphery.

ENT/OPTHALMOLOGY

case

Retinitis Pigmentosa

Differential

Best Disease

Choroquine Toxicity

Neuroretinitis

Toxoplasmosis

Discussion

Retinitis pigmentosa is a **slow degenerative disease** of the retina that is always bilateral, begins in childhood, and results in blindness by middle or advanced age; the degeneration primarily affects the rods and the cones, particularly the rods, and commences in a zone near the equator, spreading both anteriorly and posteriorly. The condition may be associated with Laurence–Moon–Biedl syndrome (characterized by obesity, hypogenitalism, and mental subnormality), Refsum's disease (peripheral neuropathy, cerebellar ataxia, deafness, and ichthyosis due to a defect in phytanic acid metabolism), and abetalipoproteinemia. The condition is inherited as an autosomal-recessive trait in 40% of cases, as autosomal-dominant in 20%, and as X-linked in 5%.

Treatment

No satisfactory treatment; genetic counseling for prevention of the disease if the pattern of inheritance in a particular family can be traced.

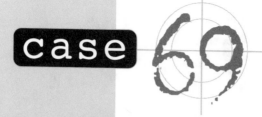

case 69

ID/CC	An **18-month-old** boy presents with **diminished visual acuity** and a wandering right eye that his mother noticed while watching him play with his toys.
HPI	On directed history, the child admits to having **eye pain** at night.
PE	**White pupillary or "cat's eye" reflex** in right eye (LEUKOCORIA); deviation of right eye (STRABISMUS); **intraocular mass** on retinal examination.
Imaging	CT/MR: orbit: lobulated, hyperdense retrolental (behind lens) mass; no optic nerve compression.
Gross Pathology	Whitish mass behind lens.
Micro Pathology	Sheets of small, round blue cells with clusters of cuboidal or short columnar cells arranged around a central lumen (FLEXNER–WINTERSTEINER ROSETTES).

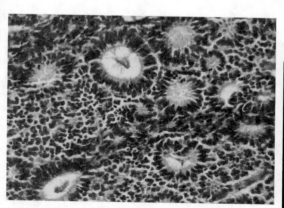

Figure 69-1. Diffuse uniform hyperchromatic cells forming rosettes.

ENT/OPTHALMOLOGY

137

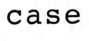

Retinoblastoma

Differential

Retinal Detachment

Cataracts

Melanoma

Retinopathy of Prematurity

Orbital Celluliti

Uveitis

Discussion

The **nonhereditary** variety of retinoblastoma appears as a single tumor; **hereditary** forms occur in early childhood and are often bilateral or multicentric. In hereditary cases, patients are at high risk for other cancers later in life (especially osteosarcoma). Cytogenetic studies reveal a **deletion on chromosome 13** (band 14 on long arm, Rb gene). Rb is a tumor suppressor gene; the loss of both allelic copies leads to malignancy (two-hit hypothesis). This important tumor suppressor gene, a nuclear phosphoprotein, normally inhibits cell cycle progression at the G1/S boundary by inhibiting the transcription factor E2F.

Treatment

Surgery; chemotherapy; radiation therapy.

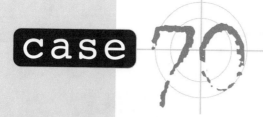
ID/CC A 30-year-old male presents with sudden-onset **pain, redness, and tearing** in his left eye.

HPI He also complains of **photophobia and blurred vision** in the left eye.

PE VS: normal. PE: ophthalmologic exam reveals **conjunctival congestion, diminished visual acuity,** normal visual field, and pupillary miosis with normal reactivity; **aqueous flare with keratic precipitates** noted in anterior chamber on slit-lamp exam.

Labs CBC: normal. ESR, ANA, RPR, VDRL, Lyme titer (to rule out systemic causes): normal.

Imaging XR: chest and sacroiliac joints: normal.

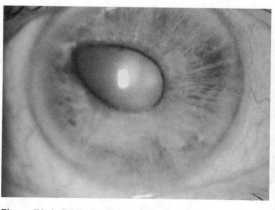

Figure 70-1. Patient's eye on presentation.

case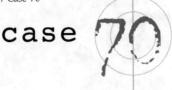

Uveitis

Differential

Conjunctivitis

Corneal Abrasion

Glaucoma

Corneal Ulceration

Keratitis

Scleritis

Discussion

Systemic disorders (sarcoidosis, SLE, ankylosing spondylitis, tuberculosis, syphilis) should be investigated as causes of uveitis.

Treatment

Cycloplegics (atropine) to relax pupillary sphincter and ciliary muscles; **topical corticosteroids;** occasionally immune suppression. Treat **underlying systemic illness.**

case 71

ID/CC A **5-year-old white** female is brought to her pediatrician because of fever, **marked weakness, pallor, bone pain,** and bleeding from her nose (EPISTAXIS).

HPI She has a history of progressively increasing fatigability and **recurrent infections** over the past few months.

PE VS: fever. PE: marked pallor; epistaxis; ecchymotic patches over skin; **sternal tenderness;** slight hepatosplenomegaly with **nontender lymphadenopathy;** no signs of meningitis; normal funduscopic exam.

Labs CBC/PBS: normocytic, normochromic **anemia; absolute lymphocytosis with excess blasts** (>30%) **and neutropenia; thrombocytopenia.** Cells are **(CALLA)** (CD10) **positive;** terminal deoxytransferase **(TDT) positive** (marker of immature T and B lymphocytes) on enzyme marker studies; negative monospot test for Epstein-Barr virus.

Imaging CXR: no lymphadenopathy.

Gross Pathology Neoplastic infiltration of lymph nodes, spleen, liver, and bone marrow with loss of normal architecture.

Micro Pathology **Myelophthisic bone marrow** (distorted architecture secondary to space-occupying lesions) with lymphoblastic infiltration; lymphoblasts with inconspicuous nucleoli, condensed chromatin, and scant cytoplasm.

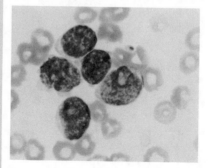

Figure 71-1. Condensed chromatin, and scant cytoplasm.

141

case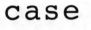

Acute Lymphoblastic Leukemia

Differential

Acute Anemia

Fanconi Anemia

Juvenile Rheumatoid Arthritis

Mononucleosis

Neuroblastoma

Non-Hodgkin Lymphoma

Parvovirus B_{19} Infection

Discussion

Acute lymphocytic leukemia (ALL) is the **most common pediatric neoplasm;** it accounts for 80% of all childhood leukemias. With treatment, it carries a **good prognosis.**

Treatment

Treat infection with antibiotics, **anemia** with blood transfusions, and **thrombocytopenia** with platelet concentrations; chemotherapy to induce, consolidate, and maintain remission; intrathecal chemotherapy and irradiation for CNS prophylaxis; bone marrow transplant during remission.

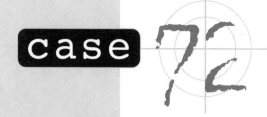

ID/CC A **25-year-old woman** presents with **high-grade fever, menorrhagia,** and marked weakness.

HPI Over the past several weeks, she has also had **recurrent infections.**

PE Marked **pallor;** multiple purpuric patches over skin; hepatosplenomegaly; **gingival hyperplasia;** sternal tenderness; normal funduscopic and neurologic exam.

Labs CBC/PBS: normocytic, normochromic **anemia; thrombocytopenia;** leukocytosis composed mainly of **myeloblasts and promyelocytes** (nonmaturing, early blast cells); **neutropenia.** Prolonged PT and PTT.

Gross Pathology Bone erosion due to **marrow expansion;** chloroma formation, mainly in skull; splenomegaly.

Micro Pathology Myeloblasts with myelomonocytic differentiation replace normal marrow (MYELOPHTHISIC BONE MARROW); **basophilic cytoplasmic bodies** (AUER RODS) in myelocytes; **peroxidase-positive** stains on bone marrow and gingival biopsy.

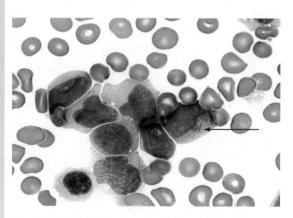

Figure 72-1. Myeloblasts and monoblasts with reddish-purple rod-shaped cytoplasmic inclusions (Auer rods).

143

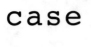

case

Acute Myelogenous Leukemia

Differential | Acute Lymphocytic Leukemia
Megaloblastic Anemia
Gaucher Disease
HIV Infection
Neuroblastoma
CMV Infection
Histiocytosis

Discussion | Acute myelogenous leukemia (AML) is not as common in children as is ALL. An increased risk is associated with ionizing radiation, benzene exposure, Down's syndrome, and cytotoxic chemotherapeutic agents. The M3 variant is associated with a t(15;17) translocation associated with the mutant expression of a retinoic acid receptor (RARα).

Treatment | Chemotherapy; all-trans retinoic acid in acute promyelocytic leukemia; bone marrow transplant during first remission if HLA-matched donor available.

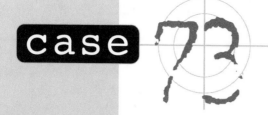

ID/CC A 12-year-old male presents with high fever, marked **pallor,** and **epistaxis;** he has a history of **recurrent URIs** and high-grade fever that have been treated with parenteral antibiotics.

HPI He has also shown **marked weakness** over the past 3 months. He lives in the vicinity of an industrial unit that handles petroleum distillates such as **benzene.**

PE VS: fever. PE: marked pallor of skin and conjunctiva; oral and nasal mucosal **petechiae; purpuric patches** visible on skin; no significant lymphadenopathy; **no hepatosplenomegaly.**

Labs CBC/PBS: **anemia, neutropenia, and thrombocytopenia** (PANCYTOPENIA); anemia with low reticulocyte count; normal RBC morphology. Normal serum bilirubin; negative Coombs' test; normal chromosomal studies.

Gross Pathology Increased yellow marrow and decreased red marrow.

Micro Pathology Hypocellular bone marrow with empty spaces populated by fat cells, fibrous stroma, and scattered lymphocytes; marked decrease in all cell lines.

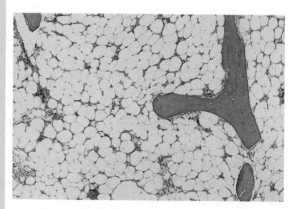

Figure 73-1. The bone marrow consists largely of fat cells and lacks normal hemopoietic activity.

145

case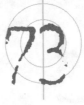

Aplastic Anemia

Differential

Acute Lymphocytic Leukemia
Acute Myelogenous Leukemia
Agnogenic Myeloid Metaplasia with Myelofibrosis
Megaloblastic Anemia
Multiple Myeloma
Myelophthisic Anemia
Non-Hodgkin Lymphoma

Discussion

Sixty-five percent of cases are **idiopathic.** Aplastic anemia following **drug or toxin exposure** may be dose dependent (e.g., benzene, cytotoxic drugs, radiation) or idiosyncratic (e.g., chloramphenicol). Other causes include **viral infection** and Fanconi's anemia, an autosomal-recessive disorder in DNA repair.

Treatment

Removal of myelotoxin (in this case, benzene); bone marrow transplantation; immunosuppressive treatment with antithymocyte globulin; myeloid growth factors (e.g., GM-CSF) for neutropenia.

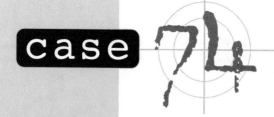

case 74

ID/CC   A 66-year-old white man recently **diagnosed with chronic lymphocytic leukemia** comes into the emergency room complaining of **fatigue** and tachycardia.

HPI   He also states that his **urine** has been progressively turning **dark and red** over the course of the day.

PE   VS: tachycardia. PE: dyspnea; pallor of skin and mucous membranes; slight jaundice; **splenomegaly.**

Labs   CBC/PBS: **severe anemia; positive direct Coombs' test (direct** antiglobulin test); **reticulocytosis;** spherocytosis; "bite cells." UA: positive for hemosiderin. Increased serum indirect bilirubin.

Gross Pathology   Congestive splenomegaly (due to **extravascular hemolysis** in the spleen).

case 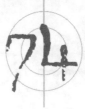 74

Autoimmune Hemolytic Anemia

Differential	Disseminated Intravascular Coagulation
	Thrombotic Thrombocytopenia Purpura
	Systemic Lupus Erythematosus
	Parvovirus B$_{19}$ Infection
	Paroxysmal Nocturnal Hemoglobinuria
Discussion	Autoimmune hemolytic anemia is idiopathic in about 50% of cases; it is characterized by autoantibodies against RBC membranes (Rh), complement activation, and phagocytosis of RBCs by splenic macrophages. Three main types exist: **warm antibody** (80% to 90%; associated with leukemia, lymphoma, SLE, and viral infections); **cold reacting antibody** (10%; associated with EBV/mycoplasma infections and lymphoma); and **drug-induced** (methyldopa, quinidine, penicillin).
Treatment	Prednisone; transfusions; splenectomy; immunosuppressive drugs. Discontinue any offending drug.

HUMAN SERUM OR
SERUM PROTEINS

ANTI IMMUNOGLOBULIN,
ANTI COMPLEMENT
ANTIBODIES PRODUCED
BY RABBIT

+

RED CELLS COATED
WITH "INCOMPLETE"
ANTIBODIES OR
COMPLEMENT

AGGLUTINATION

Figure 74-1. Rabbits or goats are immunized with human serum or serum components. The resulting sera containing anti–γ-globulin or anticomplement antibodies are then added to test samples of RBCs. If human γ-globulins, complement components, or both are bound to the cell surface, agglutination occurs.

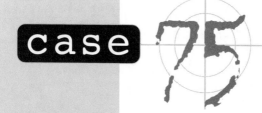

case 75

ID/CC   A 35-year-old woman is admitted to the hospital with **left-sided weakness upon awakening.**

HPI   She has **no history** of prior headaches, seizures, hypertension, or diabetes and neither smokes nor takes drugs. Her **first three pregnancies** were **spontaneously aborted;** the fourth resulted in **unexpected fetal death.**

PE   VS: normal. PE: patient conscious; mild pallor; **left hemiplegia** with exaggerated deep tendon reflexes and extensor plantar response (POSITIVE BABINSKI'S SIGN); no neck rigidity; fundus normal; no carotid bruit; no cardiac murmurs; **reddish-blue mottling of skin in fishnet pattern** (LIVEDO RETICULARIS) on extremities; positive Homans' sign in left leg.

Labs   CBC: mild thrombocytopenia. **Prolonged PTT;** normal bleeding and clotting times; **false-positive VDRL** (titer >1:18); FTA-ABS for syphilis negative; ELISA shows presence of **anticardiolipin antibody (ACA).**

Imaging   CT: head (24 hours later): hypodensity (due to infarct) in right internal capsule.

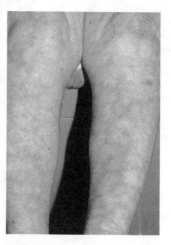

Figure 75-1. Fishnet pattern: livedo reticularis.

case

Antiphospholipid Lipid Antibody Syndrome

Differential

Bacterial Endocarditis
Mixed Connective Tissue Disease
Hepatitis B
Infectious Mononucleosis
Thrombasthenia
Rheumatic Fever

Discussion

The presence of **lupus anticoagulant** and **ACA** defines antiphospholipid syndrome; it is further characterized by **recurrent deep venous thrombosis** in the lower extremities, thrombosis in the renal and hepatic veins, **pulmonary hypertension, cerebral artery occlusion** associated with stroke and transient ischemic attacks (TIAs), and neurologic findings that resemble multi-infarct dementia or epilepsy.

Treatment

Initial therapy with heparin followed by warfarin for long-term use; low-molecular-weight heparin may be combined with aspirin for anticoagulation during pregnancy.

case 76

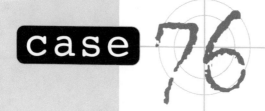

ID/CC A **9-year-old** girl, the daughter of **African** immigrants, presents with a large **swelling of the right side of her face and jaw** of 3 weeks' duration.

HPI Two weeks ago, she complained of **loosening of the** upper second left **molar**. Despite the size of the tumor, there is **no pain** associated with it.

PE Pallor; large, firm, ill-defined **mass** encompassing entire **upper mandible**, producing mild ipsilateral exophthalmos with **deformation** on right side of face.

Labs CBC/PBS: normocytic, normochromic anemia; mild leukopenia; positive direct Coombs' test. Karyotype: chromosomal translocation **t(8;14)** involving c-myc gene.

Imaging CXR: no evidence of mediastinal widening (vs. Hodgkin's lymphoma).

Gross Pathology Firm, ill-defined tumor involving upper mandible and deforming neighboring structures, but **no ulceration** or necrosis; **no satellite adenopathy.**

Micro Pathology Giemsa-stained FNA shows cells of uniform size with nongranular basophilic nuclei; **high mitotic index** and typical **"starry sky"** image pattern (due to diffuse distribution of macrophages among tumor cells).

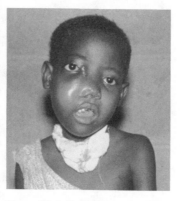

Figure 76-1. Patient on presentation.

151

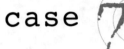 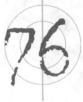

Burkitt Lymphoma

Differential

Lymphoblastic Lymphoma

Mantle Cell Lymphoma

Diffuse Large B Cell Lymphoma

Small Lymphocytic Lymphoma

Discussion

Burkitt's lymphoma is a small noncleaved lymphoma **(non-Hodgkin's lymphoma)**. It is a poorly differentiated **B-cell** lymphoblastic lymphoma. The endemic (African) form is characterized by jaw tumors and is associated with **EBV** infection; the nonendemic (Western) form is characterized by abdominal and pelvic involvement. The condition was first described by Denis Burkitt in 1958 in Uganda.

Treatment

Short-term combination chemotherapy; allopurinol and aggressive hydration with alkalinization to protect against tumor lysis syndrome; alkalinize urine, force diuresis; bone marrow transplantation for recurrent disease; intrathecal methotrexate for meningeal prophylaxis.

case 77

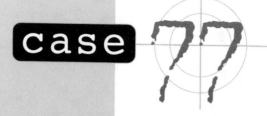

ID/CC A **65-year-old male** visits his family doctor for a routine annual checkup.

HPI On directed history, he admits to a **weight loss** of about 12 pounds over the past 4 months, together with episodes of **epistaxis** and extreme **fatigue**.

PE Generalized nontender **lymphadenopathy**; pallor; **enlargement of spleen and liver**.

Labs CBC/PBS: **markedly elevated WBC count** (124,000); **90% lymphocytes;** no lymphoblasts; mild thrombocytopenia; **Coombs-positive hemolytic anemia; smudge cells** (fragile lymphocytes). CD5 T lymphocytes on flow cytometry.

Imaging CT/US: hepatosplenomegaly.

Gross Pathology Lymph node enlargement almost always present; hepatosplenomegaly with tumor nodule formation.

Micro Pathology Bone marrow biopsy reveals extensive infiltration, mainly by normal-looking lymphocytes and a few lymphoblasts with small, dark, round nuclei and scant cytoplasm; liver, spleen, lymph node involvement common; B lymphocytes fail to mature properly.

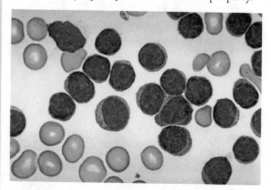

Figure 77-1. A smear of peripheral blood shows numerous small-to-medium-sized lymphocytes. A smudge cell is seen at the upper left.

153

case

Chronic Lymphocytic Leukemia

Differential

Lymphoblastic Lymphoma

Non-Hodgkin Lymphoma

Chronic Myelogenous Leukemia

Hairy Cell Leukemia

Follicular Lymphoma

Acute Myelogenous Leukemia

Discussion

Chronic lymphocytic leukemia (CLL) is a malignant neoplastic disease of **B lymphocytes** that express the surface marker CD5 (usually in T lymphocytes); it is characterized by **slow progression** of anemia, hemolytic anemia, recurrent infections, lymph node enlargement, and bleeding episodes.

Treatment

Chemotherapy; prednisone or splenectomy for complications such as autoimmune hemolytic anemia or immune thrombocytopenia.

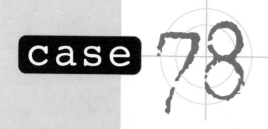

ID/CC A 40-year-old white male visits a doctor for a life insurance physical examination.

HPI The patient has no major complaints except for occasional **fatigue** and **increasing abdominal girth** (due to enlarged spleen).

PE Pallor of skin and mucous membranes; **markedly enlarged spleen; pain on palpation over sternum** (due to marrow overexpansion); no lymphadenopathy; no other abnormalities found.

Labs CBC/PBS: **markedly elevated WBC count** (130,000); immature granulocytes mixed with normal-appearing ones; **basophilia;** eosinophilia; early thrombocytosis; late thrombocytopenia. **Low leukocyte alkaline phosphatase;** elevated serum vitamin B_{12} level. Karyotype: chromosomal translocation **t(9;22)/bcr-abl gene** (PHILADELPHIA CHROMOSOME).

Imaging US: abdomen: splenomegaly.

Gross Pathology Skull chloromas (malignant, green-colored tumor arising from myeloid tissue); enlarged and congested spleen with areas of thrombosis and microinfarcts; hepatomegaly (due to proliferation and infiltration by granulocyte precursors and mature granulocytes).

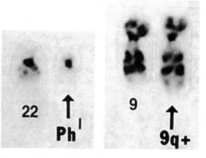

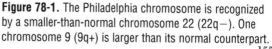

Figure 78-1. The Philadelphia chromosome is recognized by a smaller-than-normal chromosome 22 (22q−). One chromosome 9 (9q+) is larger than its normal counterpart.

case

Chronic Myelogenous Leukemia

Differential | Agnogenic Myeloid Metaplasia with Myelofibrosis
Myelodysplastic Syndrome
Myeloproliferative Disorder
Polycythemia Vera

Discussion | In chronic myelogenous leukemia (CML), death usually results from accelerated transformation into acute leukemia (BLAST CRISIS).

Treatment | Imatinib mesylate is one of the first "rationally designed drugs." It was designed specifically to inhibit the p210 gene product formed from the Philadelphia chromosome. It functions by inducing apoptosis via inhibition of tyrosine kinase in cells positive for abr-cbl; hydroxyurea; α-interferon; bone marrow transplantation.

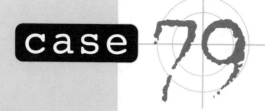

ID/CC	A 55-year-old male presents with **swelling, pain,** and **redness** of the right **leg.**
HPI	He is retired and leads a **sedentary lifestyle.** He admits to a 70-pack-year smoking history and occasional alcohol intake.
PE	VS: fever (38.4°C); tachycardia (HR 106); mild hypertension (BP 142/92); normal RR. PE: right **lower extremity swollen (>1-2 cm the contralateral leg); pain** elicited on **calf palpation** and on **dorsiflexion** of right foot (HOMANS' SIGN).
Labs	Blood **D-dimer elevated.**
Imaging	US: Doppler: **thrombi occluding right common femoral and popliteal veins.** Venography: **gold standard** for diagnosis, but rarely indicated.

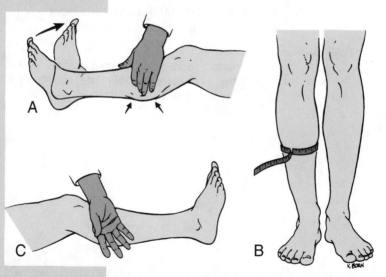

Figure 79-1. (A) Pain and tenderness in the calf of the affected extremity, especially on dorsiflexion of the foot (Homans' sign). (B) The affected extremity may have a larger circumference than the unaffected extremity, caused by edema. (C) The affected extremity will be warm to touch compared to the unaffected extremity.

case

Deep Vein Thrombosis

Differential

Baker Syndrome
Budd-Chiari
Congestive Heart Failure
Cellulitis
Superficial Thrombophlebitis

Discussion

Complications of DVT include pulmonary embolism and venous ulceration, and insufficiency. Approximately 200,000 deaths per year in the United States are attributable to pulmonary embolism secondary to DVTs.

Treatment

Anticoagulation with IV or low-molecular-weight heparin, followed by long-term anticoagulation with oral warfarin or subcutaneous low-molecular-weight heparin. Prophylaxis is commonly employed to prevent this complication in the hospital. Measures include treatment with subcutaneous heparin or the use of pneumatic compression stockings.

Breakout Point

> Virchow's triad **(venous stasis, vessel wall injury, and hypercoagulable state)** contributes to the formation of venous thrombi.

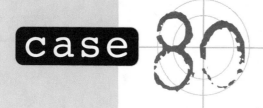

ID/CC A 25-year-old white female **continues to bleed** steadily after a normal, spontaneous vaginal delivery.

HPI Manual exploration of the uterus reveals retained placental tissue that requires dilatation and curettage; 30 minutes after the procedure, the patient begins to **bleed profusely from her gums** and continues to bleed vaginally.

PE Diffuse bleeding in gums and oral mucosa; **bleeding diathesis of skin** (both petechiae and purpura) with **oozing from venipuncture sites.**

Labs **Low fibrinogen.** CBC: **low platelet count. Prolonged PT and activated PTT; elevated fibrin degradation products,** especially D-dimers.

Gross Pathology May see complications such as renal cortical necrosis, limb thrombosis with gangrene, and ischemic adrenal necrosis.

Micro Pathology **Microthrombi** in arterioles and capillaries, leading to **microinfarcts** in practically any organ; also **hemorrhages** and petechiae in involved organs.

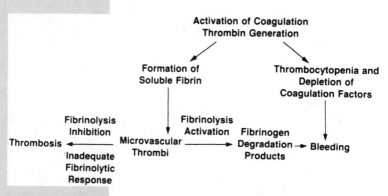

Figure 80-1. Hemorrhage and thrombosis in intravascular coagulation.

case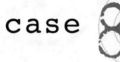

Disseminated Intravascular Coagulation

Differential
Hemolytic Uremic Syndrome (HUS)
Immune Thrombocytopenic Purpura (ITP)
Thrombotic Thrombocytopenic Purpura (TTP)
Heparin Induced Thrombocytopenia (HIT)

Discussion
Disseminated intravascular coagulation (DIC) is a bleeding disorder that is due to consumption of platelets, fibrin, and coagulation factors secondary to excessive clotting in microcirculation. It is precipitated by **cancer, gram-negative septicemia, burns,** multiple **trauma,** and **obstetric complications.**

Treatment
Treat underlying disorder; fresh frozen plasma; fibrinogen cryoprecipitate; platelets. Aggressive volume support, vasopressors.

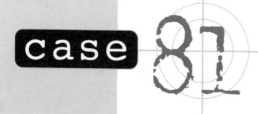

case 81

ID/CC A 35-year-old man complains of **pain in his calf muscles while walking** that is **relieved by rest** (INTERMITTENT CLAUDICATION) together with exertional chest pain.

HPI He has a family history of **premature atherosclerotic coronary artery disease (CAD)**.

PE VS: mild hypertension. PE: **obese; palmar xanthomas** and tendon xanthomas; **orange-yellow discoloration of palmar creases** (pathognomonic for **dysbetalipoproteinemia**); **tuboeruptive xanthomas** on pressure sites (elbows, buttocks, and knees); weak peripheral pulses.

Labs LFTs normal; lipid profile reveals **elevated total cholesterol, triglycerides, and VLDL and reduced LDL and HDL**; chylomicron remnants present in fasting plasma; electrophoresis reveals **beta migrating VLDL**; isoelectric focusing shows **EII/EII genotype** (nearly pathognomonic).

Imaging Angio: coronary: atherosclerotic coronary artery disease confirmed.

Gross Pathology Yellowish intraluminal atherosclerotic plaques seen in the aorta and other large vessels.

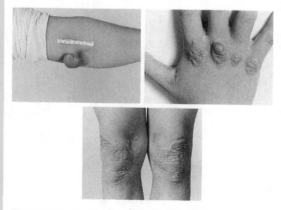

Figure 81-1. Xanthomas in familial hypercholesterolemia.

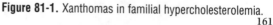

case

Dysbetalipoproteinemia

Differential

Familial Combined Hyperlipidemia

Hypothyroidism

Nephrotic Syndrome

Acute Pancreatitis

Discussion

Dysbetalipoproteinemia (TYPE III HYPERLIPOPROTEINE-MIA) is defined as the presence of **VLDL particles that migrate to the** beta **position on electrophoresis** (normal VLDL particles typically migrate to the pre-beta location). Beta-VLDL particles are chylomicrons and VLDL remnants **caused in part by a mutant apo E** that impairs the hepatic uptake of apoprotein-E-containing lipoproteins (VLDL and chylomicrons).

Treatment

Weight reduction to ideal body weight, regular exercise, **avoidance** of alcohol and other triglyceride-raising drugs; low-fat, low-cholesterol **diet;** fibric acid derivatives and niacin are drugs of choice.

case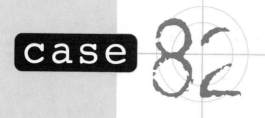

ID/CC A 61-year-old **white male** presents with marked **weakness, gingival bleeding**, and an **abdominal mass.**

HPI He has a history of **recurrent bacterial infections** and has not traveled outside the United States.

PE **Pallor; marked splenomegaly;** mild hepatomegaly; no lymphadenopathy, icterus, or ascites.

Labs CBC/PBS: **anemia; decreased WBCs and platelets** (PANCYTOPENIA); **lymphocytes with characteristic long, thin cytoplasmic projections.**

Imaging CXR: normal. CT/US: abdomen: massive splenomegaly; mild hepatomegaly; no lymphadenopathy; no evidence of portal hypertension.

Gross Pathology Liver, spleen, and bone marrow infiltrated by tumor cells.

Micro Pathology **Bone marrow largely replaced by tumor cells** (MYELOPHTHISIC BONE MARROW); large proportion of cells contain tartrate-resistant acid phosphatase **(TRAP)**; splenic biopsy reveals infiltration of red pulp by tumor cells.

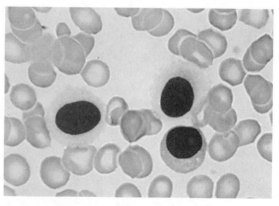

Figure 82-1. Blood smear with two "hairy" cells and a plasmacytoid lymphocyte. The cytoplasm of the hairy cells is abundant with "hairy" projections.

case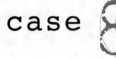

Hairy Cell Leukemia

Differential

Agnogenic Myeloid Metaplasia with Myelofibrosis
Aplastic Anemia
Chronic Lymphocytic Leukemia
Myeloproliferative Disorder
Myelodysplastic Syndrome

Discussion

Hairy cell leukemia is a very rare chronic **B-cell malignancy**; autoimmune syndromes are frequently seen, including vasculitis and arthritis. It is also characterized by **atypical mycobacterial infections.**

Treatment

2-chlorodeoxyadenosine (2-CdA) is first-line therapy; pentostatin, α-interferon, and splenectomy for selected cases.

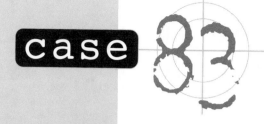

ID/CC An **8-year-old** white male presents with an erythematous skin **rash over the buttocks and legs** coupled with **joint pains, abdominal pain,** and **hematuria.**

HPI Three days before he had complained of cough, coryza, low-grade fever, and sore throat. He has a **history of allergy** to dust and pollen.

PE VS: hypertension. PE: **palpable purpuric skin lesions** over buttocks and legs; painful restriction of knee and ankle joint movement with swelling.

Labs CBC: **normal platelet count;** normal coagulation tests. Increased ESR; increased BUN and serum creatinine; elevated antistreptolysin O (ASO). UA: **RBCs and RBC casts** on urinary sediment. Positive stool guaiac test (due to occult blood); elevated serum IgA.

Gross Pathology Necrotizing vasculitis of kidneys and lungs.

Micro Pathology Renal biopsy shows focal and segmental glomerulonephritis with crescents (mesangioproliferative); **mesangial IgA deposits** on immunofluorescence.

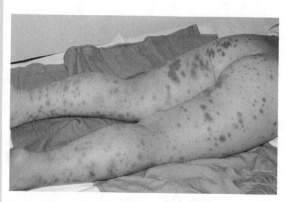

Figure 83-1. Palpable purpuric skin lesions.

case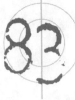

Henoch-Schönlein Purpura

Differential

Child Abuse
Bacterial Endocarditis
Meningococcal Infection
Rocky Mountain Spotted Fever
Rheumatic Fever
Systemic Lupus Erythromatosus

Discussion

Henoch-Schönlein purpura is a generally self-limited, idiopathic disorder that is also known as anaphylactoid or vascular purpura; it is a **common vasculitis (small vessel) in children.** Colicky abdominal pain is due to focal hemorrhages into the GI. Thirty percent of patients have IgA nephropathy, manifested as hematuria, proteinuria, nephrotic syndrome, mesangial immune complex deposits.

Treatment

Supportive; steroids; high-dose immunoglobulin therapy experimental; penicillin if ASO titer is elevated.

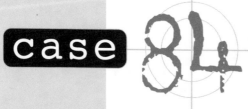

case 84

ID/CC	A **6-year-old male** is brought to a specialist by his parents due to persistent **pain and tenderness on the forehead** of a few months' duration.
HPI	There is **no history of trauma** to the affected area. The child is otherwise well and is growing normally.
PE	Exquisitely tender site found overlying forehead anteriorly; remainder of exam unremarkable.
Labs	Routine lab parameters normal.
Imaging	CXR: **punched-out lesion** of the skull.
Gross Pathology	**Intramedullary expanding, eroding lesion.**
Micro Pathology	Brownish granulation tissue containing **abundant foamy** histiocytes and **eosinophils** with leukocytes and giant cells.

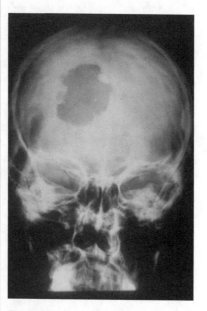

Figure 84-1. A radiograph of the skull shows a large, lytic lesion.

case 84

Histiocytosis X—Eosinophilic Granuloma

Differential

Bone Metastases

Fibrous Dysplasia

Osteomyelitis

Osteosarcoma

Bone Cyst

Discussion

Eosinophilic granuloma is a type of Langerhans cell histiocytosis; it is an indolent disorder that affects children and young adults, especially males. Solitary bone lesions may be asymptomatic or may cause pain and tenderness and, in some instances, pathologic fracture, but without any systemic manifestations. Diagnosis is based on radiographic demonstration of a localized destructive lesion arising from inside the marrow cavity. The **skull, mandible,** and **spine** are common locations. In some cases there may be spontaneous healing or fibrosis within a period of 1 to 2 years. The disease may also be multifocal, involving the lung, liver, spleen, or other organs.

Treatment

Lesions resolve spontaneously; surgical curettage may accelerate healing.

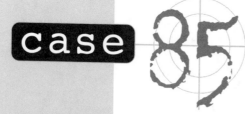

case 85

ID/CC   A 2-year-old boy is brought in for a pediatric consultation because his parents are concerned about **the child's protruding eyes** (EXOPHTHALMOS) and **excessive urine volume** (POLYURIA).

HPI   The parents also state that the child has been febrile and has had multiple ear infections.

PE   Low weight for age; bilateral exophthalmos; **painful swellings over head** (due to cystic bony lesions); no icterus; mild hepatosplenomegaly.

Labs   CBC: normal blood counts. **Increased serum osmolality; decreased urine osmolality.**

Imaging   XR: skull: **multiple rounded lytic lesions.**

Micro Pathology   Bone biopsy from skull lesions show granulomatous lesions and characteristic Langerhans cells with coffee-bean-shaped nuclei and pale, abundant cytoplasm; **tennis-racket-shaped tubular structures** (BIRBECK GRANULES) on electron microscopy; positive S-100 protein and CD1 antigen.

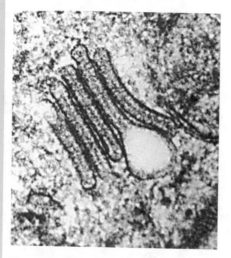

Figure 85-1. Birbeck granules.

case

Histiocytosis X—Hand-Schüller-Christian Disease

Differential

Germinoma

Sarcoidosis

Craniopharyngioma

Osteosarcoma

Ewing's Sarcoma

Discussion

A type of **Langerhan's cell histiocytosis,** Hand-Schüller-Christian syndrome is multifocal, producing **diabetes insipidus** due to the involvement of the hypothalamus and exophthalmos from orbital infiltration by histiocytes.

Treatment

Combination chemotherapy, curettage of bony lesions.

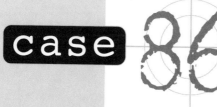

ID/CC A **2-year-old** white male child is seen with complaints of **fever** followed by a **diffuse skin rash.**

HPI The child was apparently well a month ago, born after an uncomplicated pregnancy and delivery.

PE VS: tachycardia; fever. PE: mild pallor; otoscopy of left ear reveals dull, poorly mobile tympanic membrane with pus behind it (OTITIS MEDIA); generalized lymphadenopathy; hepatosplenomegaly; diffuse maculopapular eczematous rash.

Labs CBC: anemia; thrombocytopenia with leukopenia (PANCYTOPENIA); relative eosinophilia.

Imaging CT: abdomen: hepatosplenomegaly. XR: **cystic, rarefied lesions on skull and pelvis.**

Gross Pathology Skin shows presence of extensive **eczematoid rash;** large destructive bone lesions found on skull and pelvis.

Micro Pathology **Eosinophilic granulomatous lesions** in all involved organs; EM shows typical **Langerhans cells with characteristic Birbeck granules;** expressing **CD1 antigen.**

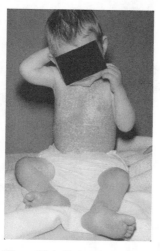

Figure 86-1. Patient (with rash) on presentation.

case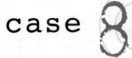

Histiocytosis X—Letterer-Siwe Disease

Differential
Immunodeficiency Syndromes
Graft versus Host Disease
Acute Leukemia
Congenital Infections
Sarcoma

Discussion
Letterer-Siwe disease is an acute or subacute clinical syndrome of unknown etiology affecting children younger than 3 years old. It is most severe form of histocytosis and is often lethal. It is marked by fever due to localized infection followed by a diffuse maculopapular eczematous purpuric skin rash and subsequent hepatosplenomegaly and generalized lymphadenopathy. It shows similarities to acute leukemia and other infectious processes. Diabetes insipidus, exophthalmos, and bone lesions are usually seen in combination.

Treatment
Corticosteroids; chemotherapy; surgery or radiotherapy for localized bone disease.

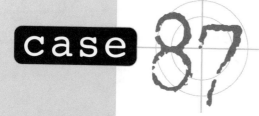

ID/CC	A **24-year-old** white **male** complains of rapid enlargement of his abdomen, producing a dragging sensation, along with a **painless lump in his neck** for the past 2 months.
HPI	The patient also complains of intermittent **fever**, drenching **night sweats**, pruritus, and **significant weight loss**.
PE	Pallor; **unilateral nontender, rubbery, enlarged cervical lymph nodes; splenomegaly;** no enlargement of tonsils.
Labs	CBC/PBS: neutrophilic leukocytosis with lymphopenia; normocytic anemia. Elevated ESR and LDH.
Imaging	CXR: **bilateral hilar lymphadenopathy.** CT, chest: mediastinal lymphadenopathy. CT, abdomen: **splenomegaly, enlarged lymph nodes,** mild hepatomegaly.
Gross Pathology	Involved lymph nodes are rubbery and have "**cutpotato**" appearance of cut surface.
Micro Pathology	Lymph node biopsy shows large histiocyte cells with multilobed nuclei and eosinophilic nucleolus resembling **owl's eyes** (REED-STERNBERG CELLS); no bone marrow involvement on bone marrow biopsy.

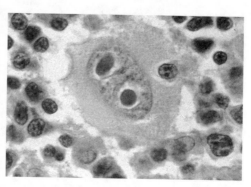

Figure 87-1. Reed-Sternberg cell.

case

Hodgkin's Lymphoma

Differential

CMV Infection
EBV Infection
Sarcoidosis
Non-Hodgkin Lymphoma
Tuberculosis
Lung Cancer

Discussion

Four patterns of Hodgkin's disease are seen on lymph node biopsy: lymphocytic predominance 5% to 10%; nodular sclerosis 65% to 75% (seen frequently in young women); mixed cellularity 20% to 30%; and lymphocyte depleted 10%. Prognosis worsens in this order. **Ann Arbor staging** I–IV with subclassification A (no constitutional symptoms) and B (weight loss, fever, night sweats) most accurately predicts prognosis. The disease **spreads to contiguous lymph nodes** before hematogenous dissemination.

Treatment

Radiotherapy and chemotherapy.

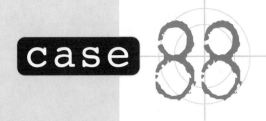

case 88

ID/CC A **3-year-old** white female is brought to the emergency room with a skin rash and **severe epistaxis**.

HPI The patient had a **URI** consisting of a severe cough and a runny nose 10 days **before the onset of her symptoms**. She has no prior history of **prolonged bleeding** following minimal trauma.

PE **Mucosal petechiae**; epistaxis; **hemorrhagic bullae** in buccal mucosa; extensive purpuric skin rash; spleen nonpalpable.

Labs CBC: mild anemia; **low platelet count** (10,000); **RBCs and WBCs normal**. Prolonged bleeding time; normal PTT; normal PT; antiplatelet antibodies detected in serum.

Gross Pathology **Purpura** (due to extravasation of blood from intravascular space into skin); pin-sized hemorrhages (PETECHIAE); ecchymosis (larger than purpura).

Micro Pathology Normal bone marrow aspirate with **increased number of megakaryocytes**.

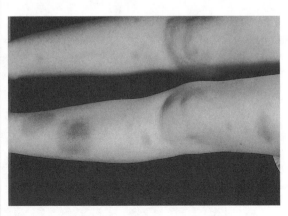

Figure 88-1. Ecchymoses of the lower extremities.

case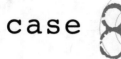

Idiopathic Thrombocytopenia Purpura

Differential
Disseminated Intravascular Coagulation (DIC)
HIV Infection
Acute Leukemia
Sepsis
Liver Disease
Pregnancy Associated Thrombocytopenia

Discussion
Idiopathic thrombocytopenic purpura (ITP) is an **autoimmune** disease with formation of **IgG antiplatelet antibodies** and subsequent platelet destruction in the spleen. It often **follows a viral infection** and is self-limited in children but chronic in adults.

Treatment
Prednisone; splenectomy; IVIG.

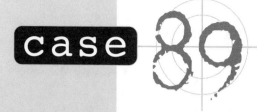

case 89

ID/CC   A **64-year-old black** male suffers from **bone pain**, weight loss, and **easy fatigability.**

HPI   He also complains of **recurrent URIs** and frequent nosebleeds.

PE   Pallor; **bone tenderness** in lower back and ribs; petechiae on buccal mucosa; no hepatosplenomegaly.

Labs   CBC/PBS: **normocytic, normochromic anemia;** neutropenia; **rouleau formation** (RBCs adhering together like a stack of poker chips). **Elevated serum calcium;** normal alkaline phosphatase; markedly **increased ESR; gamma spike on serum protein electrophoresis (monoclonal** gammopathy). UA: **Bence Jones proteinuria** (due to IgG light chains).

Imaging   XR: plain: **punched-out, lytic bone lesions** in vertebrae, long bones, and skull (axial skeleton).

Gross Pathology   Multifocal replacement of normal bone tissue with tumor cells (plasmacytoma); pelvis, skull, and spine most affected.

Micro Pathology   Infiltration of bone marrow by normal-looking plasma cells.

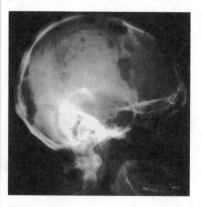

Figure 89-1. A radiograph of the skull shows numerous punched-out radiolucent areas.

177

case

Multiple Myeloma

Differential

Monoclonal Gammopathy of Unknown Significance (MGUS)

Waldenstrom Hypergammaglobulinemia

Chronic Lymphocytic Leukemia

Metastatic Cancer

Acute Lymphocytic Leukemia

Discussion

Multiple myeloma is a **primary malignancy of plasma cells** with replacement of normal bone marrow; it is the most common primary cancer in the bone. **Amyloid deposits** in kidney **(myeloma kidney)** occur with renal tubular cast formation and interstitial fibrosis (can cause **renal insufficiency**). Deposition of amyloid in the heart can cause constrictive cardiomyopathy. The prognosis worsens with anemia, renal failure, and multiple lytic lesions.

Treatment

Chemotherapeutic regimen; hydration; treat hypercalcemia and hyperuricemia; consider palliative radiation therapy; allogeneic bone marrow transplantation in selected cases. Recently a new agent bortezomib, a proteosome inhibitor, has been used as second line treatment.

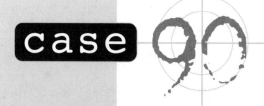

ID/CC A 54-year-old white male complains of **easy fatigability,** shortness of breath, headache, and lightheadedness over the course of almost one year, with increasing severity.

HPI He has also noticed a feeling of heaviness in his abdomen and **increasing girth** as well as recurrent deep pain in the legs and occasionally in the upper abdomen.

PE **Massive splenomegaly;** enlarged liver; moderate amount of ascitic fluid; multiple petechiae on thorax and extremities; **no lymphadenopathy.**

Labs CBC/PBS: anemia (Hb 7.2); **low hematocrit;** anemia; immature WBCs and normoblasts seen simultaneously (LEUKOERYTHROBLASTIC SMEAR); **teardrop-shaped RBCs;** giant abnormal platelets.

Gross Pathology **Extramedullary hematopoiesis,** which is prominent in liver and spleen, with significant increase in size and weight together with firm consistency.

Micro Pathology Hypocellular bone marrow (hypercellular early in disease); significant increase in number of megakaryocytes; replacement of marrow tissue with fibrosis (positive reticulin on silver stain).

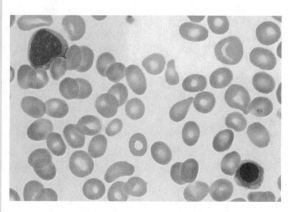

Figure 90-1. Teardrop red blood cells.

case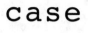

Myelofibrosis with Myeloid Metaplasia

Differential

Chronic Myelogenous Leukemia

Hairy Cell Leukemia

Myelodysplastic Syndrome

Polycythemia Vera

Essential Thrombocytosis

Discussion

Also called agnogenic myeloid metaplasia, myelofibrosis with myeloid metaplasia is an idiopathic condition in which increased secretion of platelet-derived growth factor (PDGF) and TGF-β causes **replacement of bone marrow tissue with fibrosis.**

Treatment

Transfusions; androgens; α-interferon; splenectomy; allogeneic bone marrow transplantation in younger patients.

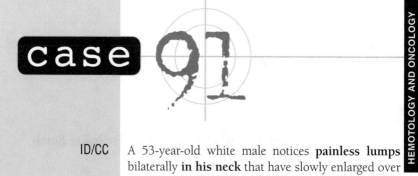

case 91

ID/CC	A 53-year-old white male notices **painless lumps** bilaterally **in his neck** that have slowly enlarged over the past 3 months.
HPI	Although he denies any pain, he admits to having episodes of mild **fever, night sweats,** and some **weight loss** over this period.
PE	Bilateral cervical **firm lymphadenopathy;** pallor; splenomegaly.
Labs	CBC: Coombs-positive hemolytic **anemia;** thrombocytopenia. **Elevated serum LDH** (a useful prognostic marker); hypogammaglobulinemia.
Imaging	CT/US: lymphadenopathy; splenomegaly.
Gross Pathology	Lymph nodes have grayish hue on outside and "**cutpotato**" appearance of cut surface.
Micro Pathology	Lymph node biopsy demonstrates nodular (well-differentiated) architecture with angulated groove cells (buttock cells).

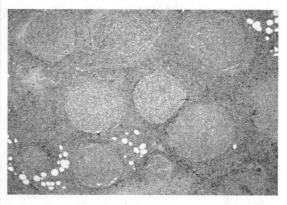

Figure 91-1. The lymph nodal architecture is replaced by homogeneous nodular aggregates of neoplastic B lymphocytes.

case 91

Non-Hodgkin's Lymphoma—Follicular Small Cleaved

Differential

Infectious Mononucleosis

Hodgkin Disease

Sarcoidosis

Metastatic Cancer

Cat-scratch Disease

Discussion

Primary malignant neoplasms of lymphocytes arise in lymphoid tissue anywhere in the body; they occur mainly in lymph nodes but may involve intra-abdominal organs and bone marrow. The prognosis is more dependent on grade than on stage. Follicular (B cell) lymphomas are the most common form and are associated with t(14;18) of bcl-2 (an anti-apoptosis protein). HIV patients have a higher incidence of non-Hodgkin's lymphoma.

Treatment

Alkylating agents in various combinations; radiotherapy if localized; bone marrow transplantation. Many B cell neoplasms, which express the antigen CD-20, are treated with the monoclonal antibody Rutuximab in addition to chemotherapy regiments like (cyclophosphamide, hydroxydaunomycin, Oncovin (vincristine), and prednisone) CHOP.

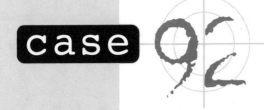

ID/CC A **62-year-old** Jewish **male** visits his family doctor because of **epistaxis**, headache, and dizziness.

HPI The patient had **black, tarry stools** (MELENA) 2 months ago and was previously admitted to the hospital for **deep venous thrombosis.** He also describes episodes of severe generalized **itching** (PRURITUS).

PE VS: **hypertension** (BP 170/100). PE: obese and **plethoric**; mild cyanosis; **palpable spleen.**

Labs CBC/PBS: **markedly increased RBC count, hemoglobin level, and hematocrit;** WBCs and platelets also increased; RBC morphology normal. Normal Po_2, Pco_2, and PT; **decreased erythropoietin level.**

Gross Pathology **Increased blood volume and viscosity** (RBC **sludging** and thrombus formation mainly in heart and brain); subnormal platelet function (bleeding tendency); increased frequency of peptic ulceration.

Micro Pathology Bone marrow biopsy shows **increase in erythroid series precursors** and, to a lesser extent, in megakaryocytes and WBC precursors.

case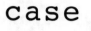

Polycythemia Vera

Differential

Chronic Myelogenous Leukemia
Secondary Polycythemia
2,3- Bisphosphoglycerate Deficiency
Essential Thrombocythemia
Myelofibrosis

Discussion

Polycythemia is characterized by an increase in RBC mass with increased blood volume and viscosity; it may be primary (polycythemia vera) or secondary (due to COPD, smoking, obesity, etc.). Decreased erythropoitein levels distinguishes polycythemia vera from secondary polycythemia. Polycythemia vera may progress to chronic myelogenous leukemia, myelofibrosis, or acute myelogenous leukemia. Patients are predisposed to thrombotic events like Budd-Chiari syndrome (hepatic vein thrombosis).

Breakout Point

> The 3 main malignancies that cause massive splenomegaly include: chronic myelogenous leukemia, polycythemia vera, and myelofibrosis with myeloid metaplasia.

Treatment

Phlebotomy; hydroxyurea; treat hyperuricemia; splenectomy in selected cases.

case 93

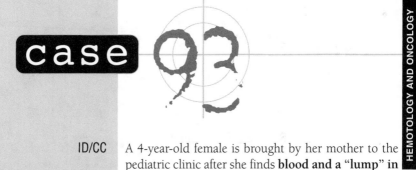

ID/CC   A 4-year-old female is brought by her mother to the pediatric clinic after she finds **blood and a "lump" in the child's vagina.**

HPI   The child's father died of brain cancer, and her mother is receiving treatment for breast cancer. Her grandfather died of metastatic colorectal cancer.

PE   Pelvic exam reveals **ulcerated, polypoid, grape-like mass** arising from wall of vagina.

Labs   Routine lab work on urine, blood, and stool yields no pathologic findings.

Gross Pathology   Bulky tumor mass with multilobed papillary projections resembling mass of grapes.

Micro Pathology   Biopsy of mass shows **desmin- and myoglobin-positive** (muscle tumor), elongated rhabdomyoblasts with large eosinophilic cytoplasm, and **cross-striations.**

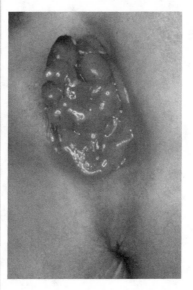

Figure 93-1. The grape-like tumor protrudes through the introitus.

185

case 93

Sarcoma Botryoides

Differential
Vaginal Polyp
Uteterocele
Hydrocolpos
Urethral Prolapse
Periurethral Cyst

Discussion
Sarcoma botryoides is a polypoidal subtype of **embryonal rhabdomyosarcoma** that characteristically protrudes like a mass of grapes from the vagina or bladder; it is the most common sarcoma in children. Rhabdomyosarcomas are often found in **"cancer families"** (e.g., Li–Fraumeni syndrome).

Treatment
Surgical resection with adjuvant chemotherapy, radiotherapy.

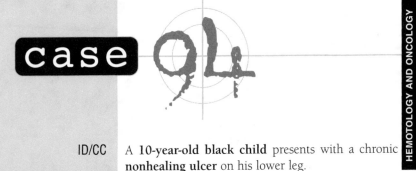

case 94

ID/CC A **10-year-old black child** presents with a chronic **nonhealing ulcer** on his lower leg.

HPI He has had recurrent episodes of **abdominal and chest pain** (due to microvascular occlusion) along with **diminution of vision**. His maternal cousin suffers from a blood disorder.

PE VS: fever. PS: **pallor; mild icterus;** funduscopy reveals **hypoxic spots with neovascularization** (SEA FANS); nonhealing chronic ulcer on left lower leg.

Labs CBC/PBS: decreased hematocrit; megaloblastic anemia; **curved RBCs; Howell–Jolly bodies and Cabot rings.** Serum bilirubin moderately elevated; quantitative hemoglobin electrophoresis shows **85% sickle cell hemoglobib (HbS).** UA: microscopic hematuria.

Imaging CT/US: abdomen: **small, calcified spleen.**

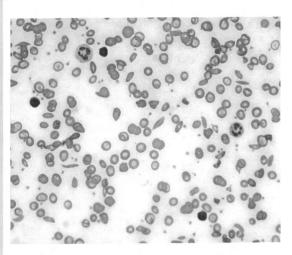

Figure 94-1. Peripheral blood smear from patient

case 94

Sickle Cell Anemia

Differential

Hemoglobin SC Disease

Hemoglobin H disease

3-beta-hydroxysteroid Dehydrogenase Deficiency

Chronic Anemia

Discussion

Sickle cell anemia is caused by a **point mutation** on the gene coding for the β chain of hemoglobin; it shows **autosomal-recessive inheritance.** Glutamic acid is substituted by valine at position 6, leading to chronic hemolytic anemia. In the reduced form, HbS forms polymers that damage the RBC membrane. Factors that hasten sickling include acidosis and hypoxemia. Prenatal diagnosis is available for at-risk fetuses.

Treatment

Local therapy for leg ulcer; laser therapy for proliferative retinopathy; antibiotic prophylaxis against capsulated bacteria; folic acid supplementation; **hydroxyurea** may help increase fetal hemoglobin levels; bone marrow transplantation.

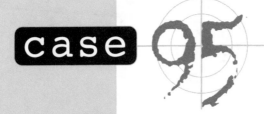
ID/CC An 11-month-old female male presents with marked **pallor, failure to thrive, and delayed developmental motor milestones.**

HPI The child's parents are **Italian** immigrants.

PE Marked pallor; mild icterus; frontal bossing and **maxillary hypertrophy** (CHIPMUNK FACIES); **splenomegaly.**

Labs CBC: severe microcytic, hypochromic anemia with **anisopoikilocytosis;** decreased reticulocytosis. **HbA absent; HbF 95%;** mildly increased unconjugated bilirubin.

Imaging XR: skull (lateral): maxillary overgrowth and widening of diploic spaces with **"hair on end" appearance** of frontal bone, caused by vertical trabeculae.

Gross Pathology Expansion of hematopoietic bone marrow, causing thinning of cortical bone or new bone formation.

Micro Pathology Red marrow increased; yellow marrow decreased; marked erythroid hyperplasia in marrow (ineffective erythropoiesis).

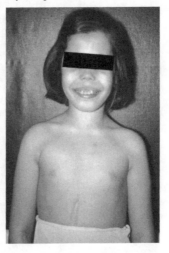

Figure 95-1. Typical chipmunk facies.

189

case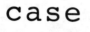

Thalassemia—Beta

Differential | Chronic Anemia
Hydrops Fetalis
Pyruvate Kinase Deficiency
Thalassemia—α
Sideroblastic Anemia

Discussion | Beta-thalassemia results from decreased synthesis of β-globin chains due to errors in the transcription, splicing, or translation of mRNA. Alpha-thalassemia results from decreased synthesis of α-globin chains due to deletion of one or more of the four α genes that are normally present.

Treatment | **Blood transfusion, folic acid supplement, iron chelation therapy** with desferrioxamine to reverse hemosiderosis, splenectomy, and **bone marrow transplantation** using HLA-matched sibling donors.

case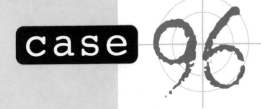

ID/CC A 23-year-old white **female** diagnosed 2 years ago as **HIV positive** is brought to the emergency room by her husband because of tachycardia, shortness of breath, headache, **intermittent disorientation,** and aphasia.

HPI She had started prophylactic **TMP-SMX** 3 weeks ago. Her husband also points out a **generalized red rash** all over her body.

PE VS: tachycardia; **fever.** PE: pale skin and mucous membranes; **confusion** and apathy **with lucid periods; petechiae** on chest and extremities; positive Babinski's sign.

Labs CBC/PBS: striking **reticulocytosis** and **fragmented RBCs** (SCHISTOCYTES); **low platelet count** (50,000); negative Coombs' test. **Absent haptoglobin; normal coagulation tests; elevated LDH.**

Gross Pathology Thrombus formation in several organs with platelet depletion and microangiopathic hemolytic anemia; kidney, brain, and heart most affected by thrombosis.

Micro Pathology Multiple hyaline thrombi in brain, myocardium, renal cortex, adrenals, and pancreas.

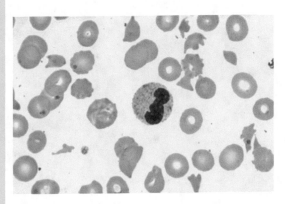

Figure 96-1. Fragmented erythrocytes (schistocytes) are seen in the blood smear.

191

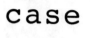

Thrombotic Thrombocytopenic Purpura

Differential

Anterior Circulation Stroke

Migraine

Complex Partial Seizure

Sepsis

Rocky Mountain Spotted Fever

Brucellosis

Discussion

Also known as Moschcowitz's syndrome, thrombotic thrombocytopenic purpura (TTP) is an idiopathic disease found in **pregnant** and **HIV positive** patients and following exposure to drugs such as **antibiotics** and **estrogens**.

Treatment

Plasmapheresis and fresh frozen plasma exchange; prednisone; splenectomy.

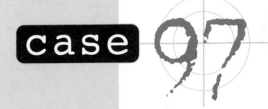

case 97

ID/CC An 18-year-old hospitalized male complains of **fever, nausea, vomiting,** and chest pain following a blood transfusion.

HPI He was involved in a motorcycle accident and was rushed to the emergency room, where he **received five units of blood** before being taken to the OR for repair of a ruptured spleen and liver.

PE VS: **fever.** PS: no hepatosplenomegaly or lymphadenopathy; surgical laparotomy wound unremarkable.

Labs **Positive Coombs' test** (indicating autoantibodies to RBCs); decreased serum haptoglobin; elevated indirect bilirubin; **cola-colored urine** (due to hemoglobinuria).

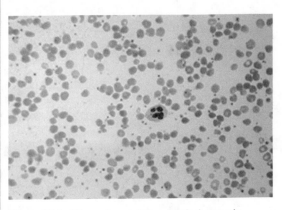

Figure 97-1. Microspherocytes and polychromasia.

193

case 97

Transfusion Reaction—Acute Hemolytic

Differential

Disseminated Intravascular Coagulation
Pulmonary Edema
Hemorrhagic Shock
Acute Cold Agglutinins
Septic Arthritis

Discussion

Acute hemolytic transfusion reaction may be the result of complete complement activation; most commonly it is a result of **mismatched blood,** producing **intravascular hemolysis.** If severe, renal shutdown or disseminated intravascular coagulation (DIC) may occur.

Treatment

Hydration; force diuresis with mannitol or furosemide; hydrocortisone; alkalinize urine with HCO_3.

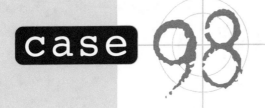

case 98

ID/CC   **During the administration of a blood transfusion,** a 45-year-old male presents with **fever, headache, and facial flushing.**

HPI   An hour later he develops **frank rigors.** He has received **several transfusions in the past,** all of which were uneventful. The last one was **a few weeks ago.**

PE   VS: fever; BP normal; tachycardia. PE: marked pallor; facial flushing; no cyanosis, icterus, or respiratory distress evident.

Labs   CBC/PBS: **negative direct and indirect Coombs' test.** Normal serum bilirubin; no incompatibility found on repeat cross-matching of donor serum and patient's blood.

case 98

Transfusion Reaction—Febrile Nonhemolytic

Differential

Anaphylaxis

Angioedema

Urticaria

Sepsis

Discussion

Febrile nonhemolytic transfusion reaction is caused by **preformed leukoagglutinins** (cytotoxic antibodies) developed after previous transfusions; it is primarily a **type II hypersensitivity reaction.** Skin rash and pruritus or anaphylaxis occur in allergic reactions mediated by IgE (due to a **type I hypersensitivity reaction**).

Treatment

Supportive; antipyretics; **leukocyte-deplete future transfusions** by filtration.

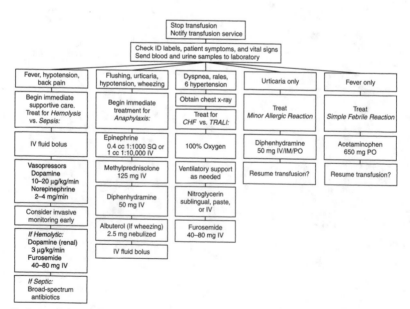

Trali=transfusion-related acute lung injury.

Figure 98-1. Clinical algorithm for suspected transfusion reaction.

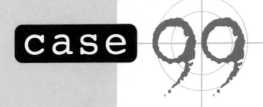

case 99

ID/CC   A 12-year-old white female is brought to the emergency room because of **uncontrollable bleeding following a tooth extraction.**

HPI   She has a **history of prolonged bleeding** following minimal trauma. Her **father** also has a **bleeding disorder.**

PE   Mucosal petechiae; epistaxis.

Labs   **Prolonged bleeding time;** normal platelet count; moderately **prolonged PTT; normal PT; quantitative assay for factor VIII reduced;** subnormal platelet aggregation in response to ristocetin; low von Willebrand's factor (vWF) antigen levels; low vWF activity.

case 99

von Willebrand's Disease

Differential Hemophilia A
Hemophilia B
Bernard-Soulier Syndrome
Antiplatelet Drug Ingestion
Platelet Function Defect

Discussion A common congenital disorder of hemostasis, von Willebrand's disease is also called vascular hemophilia. Types I and II are **autosomal dominant**; vWF factor is necessary for platelet adhesion.

Treatment Desmopressin, virally attenuated vWF concentrate (Humate-P); avoid aspirin.

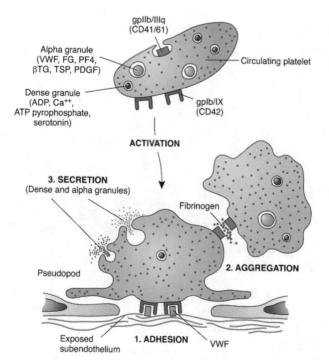

Figure 99-1. The central role of von Willebrand factor (vWF) in platelet adhesion.

case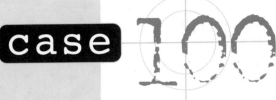

ID/CC   A **68-year-old** white male visits his doctor complaining of **weight loss**, increasing **fatigue, weakness,** headache, and **visual disturbances** over the past several months.

HPI   He also complains of **easy bruising** and **bleeding gums** while brushing his teeth.

PE   Generalized **lymphadenopathy; engorgement of retinal veins** with hemorrhages; moderate hepatosplenomegaly.

Labs   CBC/PBS: **anemia** (Hb 7.3); RBC **rouleaux formation. IgM paraprotein** (monoclonal spike on serum protein electrophoresis); increased serum viscosity. UA: normal.

Imaging   XR: plain: **absence of lytic lesions.**

Micro Pathology   Lymph node biopsy may be labeled pleomorphic lymphoma; bone marrow and spleen typically infiltrated with plasma cell precursors (plasmacytic lymphocytes); may show cytoplasmic eosinophilic, PAS-positive inclusion bodies (DUTCHER BODIES).

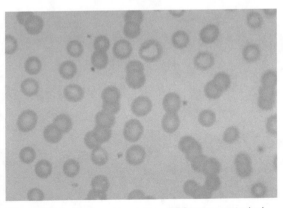

Figure 100-1. Rouleaux formation, RBCs appear stacked like poker chips.

case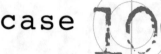

Waldenström's Macroglobulinemia

Differential

Monoclonal Gammopathy of Unknown Significance
Multiple Myeloma
Non-Hodgkin Lymphoma
Chronic Lymphocytic Leukemia
Light Chain Disease

Discussion

Waldenström's macroglobulinemia is a malignant B-lymphocyte disorder characterized by **excessive IgM** (macroglobulin) **production** and **hyperviscosity syndrome.** The sluggish blood flow results in dilation of retinal vessels and possible neurological events, TIA versus stroke. The binding of clotting factors to large amounts of serum IgM results in bleeding defects.

Treatment

Plasmapheresis (particularly with threatening vision loss); chlorambucil; cyclophosphamide; cladribine; autologous stem cell transplantation.

questions

1. A 67-year-old retired naval shipyard worker complains to his family physician about increasing shortness of breath. A chest x-ray demonstrates interstitial infiltrates. Upon referral to a pulmonologist, he undergoes a bronchoscopy that reveals ferruginous bodies. Given the patient's presentation, his likely diagnosis is:

   A. Asthma
   B. ARDS
   C. Atelectasis
   D. Fat embolism
   E. Asbestosis

2. A 23–year-old African-American female presents with fever, dyspnea, arthralgias, and tender nodules on her extremities. After an extensive workup, all of which is negative, a diagnosis of sarcoidosis is made. Of all the listed findings, which is the most likely finding in sarcoidosis?

   A. Egg shell calcifications of lymph nodes
   B. Charcot–Leyden crystals
   C. An increased Reid index
   D. Noncaseating granulomas
   E. Hyaline membrane formation

3. A 23-year-old nonsmoking female presents with shortness of breath. She has no previous medical history. A CT scan demonstrates diffuse of areas of infiltrates. A thoracic surgeon performs an open lung biopsy that demonstrates tumor cells that are proliferating along alveolar cells. This presentation is most common in which of the following lung tumors?

   A. Bronchoalveolar carcinoma
   B. Mesothelioma
   C. Small cell carcinoma
   D. Squamous cell carcinoma
   E. Bronchial carcinoid

4. A 56-year-old smoker is admitted for shortness of breath. A large left upper lobe mass is present on the chest x-ray. His laboratory results suggest a dramatically elevated calcium level. The clinical picture is suspicious for squamous cell carcinoma of the lung with the patient's hypercalcemia attributed to elevation of which substance?

    A. ACTH
    B. Autoantibodies to calcium channel receptors
    C. PTrP
    D. Serotonin
    E. ADH

5. A 13-year-old slender male complains of sudden extreme shortness of breath and chest pain while playing soccer. He is taken to the emergency room where decreased breath sounds are appreciated on the left side. A chest tube is immediately placed and the symptoms are relieved. If a chest x-ray would have been performed, what would it have shown?

    A. A thin line parallel to the chest wall representing the pleural lung
    B. A hyperinflated chest with flattening of the diaphragm
    C. Shifting of the mediastinum
    D. Honeycombing of the lung parenchyma
    E. Bilateral hilar lymphadenopathy

6. A 19-year-old female without a family history of cancer becomes obsessed with a painless mobile mass she palpates in the outer quadrant of her right breast. Clinical breast exam reveals a small, rubbery, freely mobile mass. An ultrasound of the mass demonstrates a well circumscribed mass. A core biopsy is likely to reveal which diagnosis:

    A. Fat necrosis
    B. Paget's disease of the left breast
    C. Intraductal papilloma
    D. Inflammatory carcinoma
    E. Fibroadenoma

7. A 56-year-old female is found to have a spiculated mass with an architectural distinction on a mammogram. She opts for a partial mastectomy followed by radiation therapy. She visits an oncologist following her treatment, who tells her which of the following is likely a good prognostic factor:

    A. Aneuploid tumor cells
    B. Overexpression of Her2/Neu
    C. Lymphatic invasion
    D. Estrogen progesterone receptor expression
    E. A positive family history

8. A 38-year-old African-American female reports a several year history of menorrhagia and dysmenorrhea. A complete blood count reveals the patient has iron deficiency anemia. A pelvic exam reveals a palpably enlarged uterus. What is the likely cause of the patient's dysmenorrhea?

    A. Endometrial carcinoma
    B. Primary dysmenorrhea
    C. Uterine leiomyoma
    D. Endometriosis
    E. Uterine leiomyosarcoma

9. A 33-year-old female presents to the obstetrician for an inability to conceive despite engaging in unprotected intercourse with her husband for six years. She is mildly obese and hirsute. She admits to irregular menses and is found to have a 2:1 ratio of her LH: FSH. Which of the following is likely a cause of this patient's infertility?

    A. Turner's syndrome
    B. Sheehan syndrome
    C. Polycystic ovarian syndrome
    D. Endometriosis
    E. Pre-eclampsia

10. A 23-year-old female undergoes an emergency cesarean section for a breech presentation. Following the surgery, she is transferred to the postpartum floor and found to have developed a low grade fever. Physical examination demonstrates her left calf to be swollen and painful. Doppler ultrasound of her extremity confirms the presence of a deep vein thrombosis (DVT). Which of the following could have contributed to this complication?

    A. Early ambulation
    B. Heparin used postoperatively
    C. Incentive spirometry
    D. Factor V Leyden
    E. von Willenbrand deficiency

11. A 24-year-old female presents to the emergency room with right lower quadrant pain. The patient had an appendectomy at the age of 8, and is currently menstruating. Her β-hcg is negative. A CT scan of the pelvis demonstrates an irregular calcified mass in the right lower quadrant. Which of the following is the most likely diagnosis?

A. Ovarian teratoma
B. Endometriosis
C. Ectopic pregnancy
D. Desmoid tumor
E. Stroma Ovari

12. An obese 19-year-old female presents with headaches and vision changes. Her only daily medication is oral contraceptives, and she takes NSAIDs as needed for headaches. Her ophthalmic examination reveals papilledema. Which of the following is likely in this patient?

A. Retinoblastoma
B. Acute closed angle glaucoma
C. Retinitis pigmentosum
D. Presbyopia
E. Pseudotumor cerebri

13. A 21-year-old female presents with hemoptysis and vaginal bleeding. The patient denies ever having had intercourse. Her β-hcg is markedly elevated; however, her uterus is not enlarged. A CXR shows multiple lesions in the lungs. Choriocarcinoma, a germ cell neoplasm of the ovary is suspected. Which of the following ovarian tumors is also derived from germ cells?

A. Sertoli Leydig tumor
B. Fibroma
C. Dysgerminoma
D. Brenner tumor
E. Serous cystadenocarcinoma

14. A 4-year-old child presents with weakness and pallor. She has had numerous nose bleeds over the last month. A complete blood count is performed demonstrating anemia, a dramatically elevated white blood cell count with mostly lymphocytes and a few neutrophills, as well as decreased platelets. A diagnosis of acute lymphocytic leukemia is associated with which marker?

A. CA-125
B. CALLA
C. hcg
D. Her2/Neu
E. α-antitrypsin

15. A 13-year-old is found to have decreased blood cells of all three line-
ages (red blood cells, white blood cells, and platelets) after having
numerous recurrent infections. A bone marrow biopsy is performed
revealing a hypocellular fatty marrow. He is diagnosed with aplastic
anemia, which is associated with exposure to which of the following:

A. Human papillomavirus
B. Radon
C. Chlomphenicol
D. Silicon
E. Asbestos

16. A 27-year-old male is referred to an otolaryngologist for complaints of
hearing loss and tinnitus. The patient has an MRI performed that indicates an enhancing lesion in the cerebropantine angle. A diagnosis of
acute neuroma is made. Which of the following syndromes is associated with the development of this tumor?

A. Li Fraumeni syndrome
B. Down syndrome
C. Moschcowitz's syndrome
D. Neurofibromatosis
E. Human immunodeficiency syndrome

17. A 23-year-old female presents with high grade fevers and recurrent
infections. Her complete blood count reveals anemia, thrombocytopenia with a predominance of myeloblasts, and promyelocytes.
She is diagnosed with acute myelogenous leukemia. Which is of the
following translocations can be associated with this diagnosis?

A. t(8;14)
B. t(15;17)
C. t(9;22)
D. t(14;18)
E. t(11;14)

18. An 8-year-old boy is seen in the emergency room with severe colicky
abdominal pain. On physical exam, he has a palpable purpuric lesion
on his buttocks. The patient's urinary analysis reveals hematuria. His
complete blood count is normal as are his coagulation tests. Which
of the following is the likely diagnosis?

A. Disseminated intravascular coagulation
B. Child abuse
C. Henoch–Schenlein Purpura
D. Letter–Siwe disease
E. Idiopathic thrombocytopenia purpura

19. An 18-year-old female notes enlarging supraclavicular and cervical lymph nodes. She also complains of fevers and drenching night sweats requiring her to get up and change her pajamas. A lymph node biopsy reveals Hodgkin's lymphoma. Which of the following are pathopneumonic for Hodgkin's disease?

   A. Birbeck granules
   B. Ayer rods
   C. Bence Jones proteins
   D. Reed Steinberg cells
   E. Tear drop cells

20. A 5-year-old girl is brought to the pediatrician because of a bulge of tissue protruding through the introitus of her vagina. On pelvic examination, the mass is ulcerated and polyploidy—it resembles a bunch of grapes as it arises from the lateral wall of the vagina. The physician learns that there is a strong family history of cancer. Which of the following is the most likely diagnosis?

   A. Hydatidiform mole
   B. Clear cell carcinoma of the vagina
   C. Sarcoma botroyides
   D. Vulvar leukoplakia
   E. Vulvar malignant leukoplakia

answers

1-E

    A. Asthma [incorrect] is characterized by hyperactive airways with obstruction due to bronchospasm, edema, and mucous. A chest x-ray would show hyperinflatable lungs.

    B. Acute Respiratory Distress Syndrome (ARDS) [incorrect] is a life threatening condition associated with alveolar-capillary drainage in response to a systemic condition, i.e., gram–negative sepsis or disseminated intravascular coagulation.

    C. Atelectasis [incorrect] or alveolar collapse is a common postoperative complication and is a common cause of postoperative fever.

    D. Fracture of multiple long bones, as in a motor vehicle accident, can result in a fat embolism [incorrect], which can cause hypoxia and mental status changes as small fat fragments lodge in small vessels of the lung and brain.

    E. Asbestosis [correct] exposure can result in severe parenchymal scarring decades after scar. Ferruginous bodies are asbestosis bodies coated in proteinaceous material.

2-D

    A. Silicosis, [incorrect] a form of pneumoconiosis, is associated with inhalation of silicon dust and demonstrates egg shell calcifications of lymph nodes on CXR.

    B. Charcot-Leyden crystals [incorrect] are elongated rhomboid crystals derived from eosinophil cytoplasm, found in patients with asthma.

    C. Patients with chronic bronchitis have an increase in the Reid index, [incorrect] the ratio of the mucous glands to the thickness of the bronchus.

    D. Sarcoidosis, a diagnosis of exclusion, is characterized by the presence of noncaseating granulomas [correct] in numerous tissues.

    E. Hyaline membranes [incorrect] are formed in acute respiratory distress syndrome and impede oxygenation across the alveolus, through exacerbating the cycle.

3-A

   A. Lipoic growth, growth along the alveolar walls, is pathopneumonic for broncheoalveolar carcinoma, [correct] a variant of adenocarcinoma found in young patients who do not smoke.

   B. Mesothelioma [incorrect] is a tumor of the pleural lining and is associated with smoking and asbestos exposure.

   C. Small cell carcinoma [incorrect] is closely associated with cigarette smoking. Histologically, it is characterized by small cells with scant cytoplasm.

   D. Squamous cell carcinoma [incorrect] another lung cancer closely associated with cigarette smoking is characterized by keratin pearls.

   E. Bronchial carcinoids [incorrect] are neuro-endocrine tumors that grow as fleshy polypoid masses into the bronchial lumen.

4-C

   A. ACTH [incorrect] secreted from small cell carcinomas of the lung can cause Cushing's syndrome as a paraneoplastic syndrome.

   B. Muscular weakness resembling myasthenia gravis can result from the production of autoantibodies to calcium channel receptors [incorrect] by small cell carcinoma of the lung.

   C. Parathyroid hormone related peptide [correct] produced by squamous cells in lung cancer, mimics the action of normal PTH resulting in hypercalcemia as in vignette 6.

   D. Carcinoid tumors, typically of the gastrointestinal tract, metastasize to the liver and produce serotonin [incorrect] causing diarrhea, flushing, and cardiac valve drainage in patients.

   E. Overproduction of ADH [incorrect] by small cell carcinoma of the lung can cause diabetes insipidus.

5-A

   A. A classic presentation of idiopathic spontaneous pneumothorax. The symptoms were relieved by clot placement; however, had the clinical presentation not been so obvious a CXR would have been ordered demonstrating a thin line parallel to the chest wall representing the pleural lining [correct].

   B. Patients with emphysema remain well oxygenated, "pink puffers," as they overventilate leading to a hyperinflated chest with flattening of the diaphragm [incorrect].

   C. Shifting of the mediastinum [incorrect] is rarely associated with idiopathic spontaneous pneumothorax and is more likely to occur in patients who have been mechanically ventilated [incorrect].

D. Honeycombing of the lungs [incorrect] is a chest x-ray finding in idiopathic pulmonary fibrosis.

E. Patients with sarcoidosis have characteristic bilateral hilar lymphadenopathy often referred to on the x-ray as "potato nodules" [incorrect].

6-E

A. Fat necrosis [incorrect] can present as a lump;however, it is usually painful, secondary to some antecedent trauma to the breast.

B. Paget's disease of the breast [incorrect] presents with erosion and crusting of the nipple. There is often an underlying intraductal carcinoma.

C. Intraductal papilloma of the breast [incorrect] is a benign proliferation of ductal cells within the lactiferous ducts that present with a bloody nipple discharge.

D. Inflammatory carcinoma of the breast [incorrect] presents with skin erythema and retraction of the skin leading to a "peau d'orange" appearance with or without an underlying breast mass.

E. A fibroadenoma [correct] is the most common benign breast tumor in females, especially in younger patients. It is freely mobile, typically in the lower quadrants, opposed to cancer, which is typically in the upper outer quadrant. It also varies in size with respect to estrogen level changes during the menstrual cycles.

7-D

A. In general tumors which are aneuploidal [incorrect] have a worse prognosis than those that are euploid.

B. Overexposure of the receptor tyrosine kinase Her2/neu [incorrect] is generally a poor prognostic factor; however, patients with overexpression are candidates for treatment with the therapeutic antibodies to the receptor.

C. Lymphatic invasion [incorrect] is a poor prognostic factor, suggesting that tumors have broken through the basement membrane and may gain access to a route of metastasis.

D. Patients whose tumors express estrogen and progesterone [correct] usually have a better prognosis and can be treated with hormonal therapy.

E. Although having a positive family history [incorrect] may be a risk factor for the development of breast cancer, there is no prognostic significance.

8-C

A. Endometrial carcinoma [incorrect] is a common cause of post-menopausal bleeding; however, it is unlikely to be painful.

B. Primary dysmenorrhea [incorrect] is typically seen in younger females and is thought to be due to an increase in the production of prostaglandins.

C. The most common tumors in women are uterine leiomyomas [correct]; whose growth is estrogen dependent. They frequently cause painful and heavy menstrual periods.

D. Endometriosis [incorrect] can cause dysmenorrhea as well, but there is rarely a palpably enlarged uterus. However, in cases of a chocolate cyst, the ovaries may be enlarged.

E. Uterine leiomyosarcomas are rare, malignant counterparts to a leiomyoma [incorrect].

9-C

A. Turner's syndrome [incorrect] is a major cause of amenorrhea; as such these patients are infertile. The have web necks, widely spaced nipples, and a genetic genotype of 45, XO.

B. Sheehan syndrome [incorrect] results from postpartum pituitary necrosis secondary to blood loss. These patients may experience amenorrhea and an inability to lactate.

C. Patients with polycystic ovarian syndrome [correct] present with obesity, hirsuitism, and oligomenorrhea with infertility secondary to anovulation.

D. Endometriosis [incorrect] is a leading cause of infertility; however, these patients have regular painful periods.

E. Pre-eclampsia is a condition during pregnancy associated with the development of hypertension, proteinuria, and edema that can progress to eclampsia with the development of seizures [incorrect].

10-D

A. Immobility, rather than early ambulation [incorrect], would have contributed to the development of deep vein thrombosis in this patient.

B. Anticoagulation is often given prophylactically in immobilized patients and therefore heparin [incorrect] may be used postoperatively to prevent venous thrombosis.

C. Incentive spirometry [incorrect] is indeed encouraged in postoperative patients; however, this is used to prevent atelectasis, not venous thrombosis.

D. Virchow's triad of venous stasis, vessel wall injury, and hypercoagulability all contribute to the development of deep vein thrombosis. Factor V Leyden, [correct] the most common genetic cause of hypercoagulability, indeed is a contributing factor.

E. Deficiency of von Willebrand factor [incorrect] is one of the most common congenital disorders of stasis. This defect, does not contribute to the development of deep vein thrombosis, but may actually help to prevent such a complication.

11-A

A. An ovarian teratoma, [correct] is a benign neoplasm of the ovary derived from mature tissue elements representing all three germ cell layers, including skin, neural tissue, and bone (which appears calcified).

B. Endometriosis [incorrect] can form an ovarian mass in the event that it forms a chocolate cyst within the ovaries; however, there would not be any calcifications.

C. Patients with ectopic pregnancies [incorrect] could present with right lower quadrant pain, but could likely not have a normal menstrual period and have an elevated β-hcg.

D. Desmoid tumors [incorrect] usually occur along the anterior abdominal wall and are painless, ill-defined palpable masses.

E. Stroma ovarii [incorrect] is a cystic lesion of the ovary composed of thyroid tissue.

12-E

A. Retinoblastoma [incorrect] can cause vision changes but typically in younger patients. It is a malignant tumor, which usually presents with leukouria.

B. Acute closed angle glaucoma [incorrect] can cause loss of vision and acute eye pain, although the opthalmic exam would show a hypermic and edematous optic nerve bed.

C. Retinitis pigmentosa [incorrect] results in progressively narrowing visual fields and a waxy appearance of the optic disk with narrowing and attenuation of the vessels.

D. Presbyopia [incorrect] is an age-related blurring of near vision. It is common in patients older than 45 years of age.

E. Pseudotumor cerebri [correct] can cause papilledema and progressive optic neuropathy. It occurs most commonly in obese females and is often associated with oral contraceptive use.

13-C

    A. Sertoli-Leydig tumors [incorrect] are malignant tumors derived from the epithelium of the ovary and secrete weak androgens resulting in masculinization of females.

    B. Fibromas [incorrect] are benign tumors of the gonadal stroma. Half of the large tumors are associated with ascites and pleural effusions (Meig's syndrome).

    C. Dysgerminomas [correct] are the female equivalent of seminomas in males. These are malignant tumors derived from germ cells.

    D. Brenner tumors [incorrect] are benign tumors of the epithelium of the ovary.

    E. The most common tumor of the ovary, the serous cystadenoma [incorrect], is derived from the epithelium of the ovary.

14-B

    A. Ovarian tumors are associated with an element of CA-125 [incorrect].

    B. CALLA, [correct] the most common acute lymphoblastic leukemia antigen, or CD10, is a diagnostic marker of acute lymphocytic anemia.

    C. hCG [incorrect] is produced by cells of the placenta and is elevated in normal pregnancy. It may also be found elevated in hydatidiform mole and choriocarcinoma.

    D. Her2/neu [incorrect] is overexpression in breast cancer and is often a poor prognostic indicator.

    E. Patients with a deficiency of α-antitrypsin [incorrect] are prone to the development of panacinar emphysema.

15-C

    A. Human papillomavirus (HPV) [incorrect] exposure is associated with the development of cervical cancer, especially HPV 16 and 18.

    B. Radon [incorrect] exposure is a major risk factor for the development of bronchogenic carcinoma.

    C. An idiosyncratic reaction to chloramphenicol [correct] is the development of aplastic anemia, a condition for which a bone marrow transplant is often required.

    D. Silica exposure can cause interstitial lung disease and silicosis is one of the most common pneumoconiosis [incorrect].

    E. Asbestos [correct] exposure is associated with the development of malignant mesothelioma, a tumor of the pleural lining.

16-D

A. Li-Fraumeni syndrome [incorrect] is associated with numerous cancers including those of the breast, CNS, and sarcomas. Patients have a mutation in the tumor suppressor gene p53.

B. Patients with Down syndrome [incorrect] have an increased incidence of acute leukemias.

C. Patients with the Moschowitz's syndrome [incorrect] have microangiopathic hemolytic anemia and thrombocytopenia.

D. Neurofibromatosis [correct] is a disorder due to an inherited defect in the NF-1 protein, which is usually activated by the ras-oncogene. It is a syndrome characterized by schwannomas (acoustic neuromas) and plexiform neurofibromas.

E. Patients with human immunodeficiency syndrome [incorrect] are prone to the development of numerous neoplasms, and probably lymphomas

17-B

A. t(8;14) [incorrect] is associated with Burkitt's lymphoma and results in the expression of the myc gene under the control of the Ig heavy chain promoter.

B. t(15;17) [correct] results in the formation of an aberrant retinoic acid receptor leading to aberrant cell proliferation and differentiation seen in M3 AML.

C. t(9;22) [incorrect] results in the formation of the protein tyrosine kinase bcr-abl.

D. t(14;18) [incorrect] is found in follicular lymphoma. The expression of the anti-apoptotic gene bcl-2 is dramatically increased under the control of the Ig heavy chain promoter.

E. t(11;14) [incorrect] is associated with mantle cell lymphoma with aberrant expression of cyclin D.

18-C

A. Disseminated intravascular coagulation [incorrect] often occurs in response to overwhelming sepsis and would be associated with a profound decrease in platelets as well as dramatically elevated coagulation times.

B. Although unfortunate, sometimes palpable purpura is confused with bruises inflicted as a result of child abuse [incorrect].

C. Henoch–Schenlein Purpura [correct] is a vascular disorder characterized by palpable purpura, as well as a close association with IgA nephropathy, which accounts for the hematuria.

  D. Letter–Siwe disease [incorrect] results in a diffuse skin rash and fever. This results from a defect in CD1 positive Langerhans cells.

  E. Idiopathic thrombocytopenia purpura [incorrect] can result in multiple ecchymosis and is due to antibodies to platelets that result in their destruction.

19-D

  A. Birbeck granules [incorrect] are found within CD1 positive cells of histocytosis X diseases.

  B. Ayer rods [incorrect] are basophilic cytoplasmic bodies found in the abnormal myelocytes in acute mylogenous leukemia.

  C. Bence Jones proteins [incorrect] are free light chains produced by malignant B cells of multiple myeloma.

  D. Reed Steinberg cells [correct] are large tumor cells with multi-lobed nuclei and eosinophilic nucleolus resembling owl's eyes.

  E. The characteristic cells found in myeloid metaplasia, dacrocytes, are referred to as tear drop cells [incorrect].

20-C

  A. Hydatidiform mole [incorrect] is a gestational trophoblastic disease that can cause a discharge that resembles a bunch of grapes, although it occurs as a fenestration product.

  B. Clear cell carcinoma of the vagina [incorrect] usually occurs later in life and is associated with the use of DES in mothers of affected patients.

  C. This lesion is most suspicious for an embryonal rhabdomyosarcoma of the vagina, sarcoma botryoides [correct]. It is found more commonly in families with inherited cancer syndromes.

  D. Vulvar leukoplakia [incorrect] presents as a whitish lesion on the vulva of older women. Such lesions must always be biopsied out of concern for neoplasm.

  E. Vulvar malignant leukoplakia [incorrect] is the second most common malignancy of the vulva. Again, this is more common in older patients.

credits

Anderson SC. Anderson's Atlas of Hematology. Wolters Kluwer Health/Lippincott Williams & Wilkins, 2003. (Case 72), (Case 100).

Avery GB, Fletcher MA, MacDonald MG. Neonatology: Pathophysiology and Management of the Newborn, 5th ed. Philadelphia: Lippincott Williams & Wilkins, 1999. Fig. 13.29 (Case 58).

Bailey BJ, Johnson JT, et al. Head and Neck Surgery – Otolaryngology. 4th ed. Philadelphia: Lippincott Williams & Wilkins, 2006. Figs. 50.1 (Case 63), Table 19.3 (Case 65).

Becker KL, Bilezikian JP, Brenner WJ, et al. Prinicples and Practice of Endocrinology and Metabolism, 3rd ed. Philadelphia: Lippincott Williams & Wilkins, 2001. Fig. 7.13A (Case 67).

Berek JS. Novak's Gynecology. 13th ed. Philadelphia: Lippincott Williams & Wilkins, 2002. Fig. 13.15 (Case 44).

Berek JS, Hacker NF. Practical Gynecologic Oncology. 4th ed. Philadelphia: Lippincott, Williams & Wilkins, 2004. Figs. 6.69 (Case 41), 13.10 (Case 52).

Berg D, Worzala K. Atlas of Adult Physical Diagnosis. Philadelphia: Lippincott Williams & Wilkins, 2005. Fig. 7.46 (Case 59-1).

Bhushan V, Le T, Pall V. Underground Clinical Vignettes: Step One - Pathophysiology I. 4th ed. Malden, Massachusetts: Blackwell Publishing, 2005. Figs. 010 (Case 10), 022 (Case 26), 027 (Case 31), 028 (Case 32), 031 (Case 35), 032 (Case 36), 044 (Case 48), 045 (Case 49), 065 (Case 69), 078 (Case 82), 084 (Case 88), 070 (Case 97).

Bickley LS, Szilagyi P. Bates' Guide to Physical Examination and History Taking, 8th ed. Philadelphia: Lippincott Williams & Wilkins, 2003. (Case 62).

Cagle PT. Color Atlas and Text of Pulmonary Pathology. Philadelphia: Lippincott Williams & Wilkins, 2005. Fig. 10.43 (Case 13).

Crapo JD, Glassroth J, Karlinsky JB, King TE. Baum's Textbook of Pulmonary Diseases, 7th ed. Philadelphia: Lippincott Williams & Wilkins, 2004. Figs. 44.4 (Case 2), 1.23 (Case 19), 28.2A (Case 24).

Eisenberg RL. Clinical Imaging: An Atlas of Differential Diagnosis. 4th ed. Philadelphia: Lippincott Williams & Wilkins. Figs. C28-5 (Case 21), C11-5 (Case 25), MA 4-6 (Case 27), MA 2-1 (Case 33), MA 1-2 (Case 34), SK 14-1 (Case 61).

Fleisher GR, Ludwig S, Baskin MN. Atlas of Pediatric Emergency Medicine. Phildelphia: Lippincott Williams & Wilkins, 2004. Figs. 24.1 (Case 60), 6.8B (Case 83).

Goodheart HP. Goodheart's Photoguide of Common Skin Disorders, 2nd ed. Philadelphia: Lippincott Williams & Wilkins, 2003. Fig. 25.27 (Case 75).

Goroll AH, Mulley AG. Primary Care Medicine: Office Evaluation and Management of the Adult Patient. 5th ed. Philadelphia: Lippincott, Williams & Wilkins, 2005. Fig. 212-1 (Case 65).

Greenberg MJ, Hendrickson RG. Greenberg's Text-Atlas of Emergency Medicine. Philadelphia: Lippincott, Williams & Wilkins, 2004. Fig. 7-18A (Case 55).

Greer JP, Foerster J, et al. Wintrobe's Clinical Hematology. 11th ed. Philadelphia: Lippincott Williams & Wilkins, 2003. Fig. 35.4 (Case 74).

Humes HD. Kelley's Textbook of Internal Medicine. 2nd ed. Philadelphia: Lippincott Williams & Wilkins, 2001. Figs. 179.1 (Case 12), 125.1 (Case 80).

Lee G, Foerster J, Lukens J, et al. Wintrobe's Clinical Hematology, 10th ed. Philadelphia: Lippincott Williams & Wilkins, 1998. Fig. 10.12A (Case 95).

LifeART image copyright 2006 Lippincott Williams & Wilkins. All rights reserved (Case 54).

McClatchey KD. Clinical Laboratory Medicine, 2nd ed. Philadelphia: Lippincott Williams & Wilkins, 2002. Figs. 44.25A (Case 71), 45.13 (Case 90).

McMillan JA, Fergin RD, et al. Oski's Pediatrics: Principles and Practice. 4th ed. Philadelphia: Lippincott Williams & Wilkins, 2006. Figs. 128.8 (Case 68), 314.1 (Case 86), 290.1 (Case 94).

Mulholland MW, Lillemoe KD. Greenfield's Surgery: Scientific Principles and Practice. 4th ed. Philadelphia: Lippincott Williams & Wilkins, 2005. Fig. 81.5 (Case 17).

Nettina SM. The Lippincott Manual of Nursing Practice, 7th ed. Philadelphia: Lippincott Williams & Wilkins, 2001. Fig. 14.1 (Case 79).

Rosen PP. Rosen's Breast Pathology. 2nd ed. Philadelphia: Lippincott Williams & Wilkins, 2001. Fig. 35.31 (Case 29).

Rubin E, Farber JL. Pathology, 3rd ed. Philadelphia: Lippincott Williams & Wilkins, 1999. Figs. 12.43 (Case 7), 12.49a (Case 8), 12.83a (Case 15), 12.95a (Case 18), 7.5 (Case 23), 19.4c (Case 28), 21.4 (Case 56), 20.17 (Case 73), 9.9 (Case 76), 20.57 (Case 77), 5.25c (Case 78), 10.20 (Case 81), 26.26a (Case 84), 24.5b (Case 85), 10.8 (Case 87), 20.77 (Case 89), 20.61 (Case 91), 18.10a (Case 93), 20.31 (Case 96), 20.11 (Case 99).

Rubin E, Gorstein F, Schwarting R, et al. Rubin's Pathology: A Clinicopathologic Approach. 4th ed. Baltimore: Lippincott Williams & Wilkins, 2004. Figs. 6-45 (Case 1), 12-10 (Case 5), 12-83 (Case 14), 12-82A (Case 16), 12-75A (Case 22), 19-8B (Case 30), 30-7 (Case 39), 18-67 (Case 40), 18-56B (Case 43), 18-7A (Case 51), 18-44 (Case 53), 18-73 (Case 57).

Sadler T. Langman's Medical Embryology, 9th ed. Image Bank. Baltimore: Lippincott Williams & Wilkins, 2003. 14.37 (Case 47).

Scott JR, Gibbs RS, et al. Danforth's Obstetrics and Gynecology. 9th ed. Philadelphia: Lippincott Williams & Wilkins, 2003. Figs. 55.1 (Case 45), 34.4 (Case 46), 51.5 (Case 50).

Swischuk L. Emergency Radiology of the Acutely Ill or Injured Child, 2nd ed. Philadelphia: Lippincott, Williams & Wilkins, 1986:63,77,79. Figs. 2.2A (Case 20), 2.2C (Case 4).

Tasman W, Jaeger E. The Wills Eye Hospital Atlas of Clinical Ophthalmology, 2nd ed. Philadelphia: Lippincott Williams & Wilkins, 2001. Figs. 1.39A (Case 70), 3.84 (Case 64).

Wolfson AB, Hendey GW, et al. Harwood-Nuss' Clinical Practice of Emergency Medicine. 4th ed. Philadelphia: Lippincott Williams & Wilkins, 2005. Figs. 22.1 (Case 58), 156.1 (Case 98).

case list

PULMONOLOGY

1. Acute Respiratory Distress Syndrome (ARDS)
2. Asbestosis
3. Bronchial Asthma
4. Atelectasis—Postoperative
5. Bronchiectasis
6. Churg-Strauss Syndrome
7. Chronic Bronchitis
8. Emphysema
9. Carbon Dioxide Narcosis
10. Fat Embolism
11. Hypersensitivity Pneumonitis
12. Idiopathic Pulmonary Fibrosis
13. Bronchogenic Carcinoma— Squamous Cell Carcinoma
14. Bronchogenic Carcinoma— Small Cell Carcinoma
15. Bronchogenic Carcinoma— Adenocarcinoma
16. Bronchogenic Carcinoma— Bronchoalveolar Carcinoma
17. Bronchial Carcinoid
18. Malignant Mesothelioma
19. Pleural Effusion
20. Spontaneous Pneumothorax
21. Tension Pneumothorax
22. Primary Pulmonary Hypertension
23. Pulmonary Embolism
24. Sarcoidosis
25. Silicosis

GYNECOLOGY

26. Cystosarcoma Phyllodes
27. Fat Necrosis of the Breast
28. Fibrocystic Disease of the Breast
29. Inflammatory Carcinoma of the Breast
30. Intraductal Papilloma
31. Lobular Carcinoma of the Breast
32. Paget's Disease of the Breast
33. Infiltrating Ductal Carcinoma
34. Fibroadenoma
35. Cervical Carcinoma in Situ
36. Gestational Choriocarcinoma
37. Desmoid Tumor
38. Primary Dysmennorrhea
39. Endometrial Carcinoma
40. Endometriosis
41. Hydatidiform Mole
42. Menopause
43. Serous Cystadenocarcinoma of the Ovaries
44. Ovarian Cyst—Follicular
45. Ovarian Teratoma
46. Polycystic Ovarian Syndrome
47. Primary Amenorrhea—Turner Syndrome
48. Uterine Fibroids
49. Uterine Leiomyosarcoma
50. Vulvar Carcinoma
51. Vulvar Leukoplakia

OBSTETRICS

52. Vulvar Malignant Melanoma
53. Ectopic Pregnancy
54. Postpartum Hemorrhage
55. Postpartum Thrombophlebitis
56. Sheehan's Syndrome
57. Toxemia of Pregnancy— Preeclampsia

ENT/OPTHALMOLOGY

58. Acute Closed Angle Glaucoma
59. Benign Positional Vertigo
60. Basilar Skull Fracture
61. Acoustic Neuroma
62. Labyrinthitis
63. Obstructive Sleep Apnea
64. Open Angle Glaucoma
65. Presbycusis
66. Presbyopia
67. Pseudotumor Cerebri
68. Retinitis Pigmentosa
69. Retinoblastoma
70. Uveitis

HEMOTOLOGY AND ONCOLOGY

71. Acute Lymphoblastic Leukemia
72. Acute Myelogenous Leukemia
73. Aplastic Anemia
74. Autoimmune Hemolytic Anemia
75. Antiphospholipid Lipid Antibody Syndrome
76. Burkitt Lymphoma
77. Chronic Lymphocytic Leukemia
78. Chronic Myelogenous Leukemia
79. Deep Vein Thrombosis
80. Disseminated Intravascular Coagulation

81. Dysbetalipoproteinemia
82. Hairy Cell Leukemia
83. Henoch-Schönlein Purpura
84. Histiocytosis X—Eosinophilic Granuloma
85. Histiocytosis X—Hand-Schüller-Christian Disease
86. Histiocytosis X—Letterer-Siwe Disease
87. Hodgkin's Lymphoma
88. Idiopathic Thrombocytopenic Purpura
89. Multiple Myeloma
90. Myelofibrosis with Myeloid Metaplasia
91. Non-Hodgkin's Lymphoma—Follicular Small Cleaved
92. Polycythemia Vera
93. Sarcoma Botryoides
94. Sickle Cell Anemia
95. Thalassemia—Beta
96. Thrombotic Thrombocytopenic Purpura
97. Transfusion Reaction—Acute Hemolytic
98. Transfusion Reaction—Febrile Nonhemolytic
99. von Willebrand's Disease
100. Waldenström's Macroglobulinemia

index

Page numbers followed by *f* or *t* refer to illustrations or tables, respectively.